Living On A
Roller Coaster

FOR Some... LiFe is Full oF hurts & pain,
But with God's help & Angels Like you (ACT.),
I'll bounce back once AGAin.
FoR I had my Failures, but never defeat,
Because with hearts like yours, I Feel
The Lord in The passengers seat...
    And, God AT the wheel!

James O. Wessinger III

LIVING ON A ROLLER COASTER

LIVING ON A ROLLER COASTER

The Latest Poetry Won The Golden
Poet Award International

*The Life of a
Manic-Depressive
or Biopolar Disorder.
A Manic Can Be
Very Successful,
Dynamic and Creative*

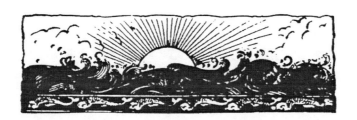

WESSINGER FOUNDATION
Thomasville Goeriga
2001

Printed in the United States of America

ISBN: 1-929925-84-0
Published & Printed by:
FirstPublish, Inc. & QUESTprint
300 Sunport Lane
Orlando, Florida 32809
http://www.firstpublish.com

To order additional copies of this book, please send $19.95, includes tax, shipping and handling. For orders of three copies or more-$17.95 each. Rush delivery with money orders.
Please send your check or money order to:

Wessinger Foundation
P.O. Box 94
Thomasville, GA   31799

TABLE OF CONTENTS

LIVING ON A ROLLER COASTER

Dedication

I would like to dedicate this book to my to numerous friends to mention, who have stood beside me, like the late attorney, Joseph Jacobs, and to the loving memory of my father, who was manic depressive and passed away in 1980. Last but no least, to my Lord and Savior, who directed me throughout this writing. Christ once said, "A man's mind leads the way, but the Lord directs him." — So true!

LIVING ON A ROLLER COASTER

INTRODUCTION

Manic depression my seem a psychological illness to many, but James 0. Wessinger III demonstrates that the manic energy it inspires can be a blessing-indeed, the secret of success. The author is a committed Christian who has learned from the Bible that this apparently debilitating affliction is in fact a gift from the Almighty shared by a surprising number of artistic geniuses, historical heroes and dynamic business leaders. Behind the astonishing achievements of such great writers as Balzac and Hemingway and such political giants as Winston Churchill, lie bouts of depression and bursts of manic energy for which Mr. Wessinger expresses great sympathy and understanding.

In his own life the author has experienced the same challenging series of ups and downs and has channelled the manic depressive's characteristic drive into productive and financially rewarding endeavors. He has also overcome a long series of obstacles and setbacks while maintaining his self-confidence and refusing to succumb to discouragement. When barely a teenager, he started up a lucrative nursery business, only to have to turn it over to his father. His manic energy, however, permitted him to carry on into even greater enterprises until he was a pillar of the community-though teetering on the precipice of a painful divorce. He dramatically describes the universality of his wins and losses, proving that manic depression and energy are not merely the preserve of the lonely few.

Wessinger knows more about the subject than many experts, in that his knowledge derives from first-hand experience of manic conditions. His seemingly interminable struggles with medical bureaucracies and mental institutions, as he is committed and released time and again without apparent justification, make for a harrowing, Kafkaesque account of a man at the mercy of the system. Still, the indefatigable Wessinger has the vision and faith not only to survive but to rise in the end, with the help of the Living Bible, to the heights of true Christian forgiveness.

The author supplements his gripping personal saga with a wealth of analysis and data concerning manic depression in general, making this an informative handbook as well as an inspirational autobiography. Throughout, the author's hard-won wisdom is founded on the precept of Christ that serves as an epigraph to *Manic Energy* and Living on a roller coaster: "A man's mind leads the way, but the Lord directs him."

LIVING ON A ROLLER COASTER

LIVING ON A ROLLER COASTER

CHAPTER I

WHAT DOES IT MEAN TO BE MANIC
OR HYPERMANIC?
SYMPTOMS AND FAMILY REACTIONS

Manic depression can without a doubt be a serious mental illness or disorder. It is, however, the easiest to treat. A manic can be more productive, dynamic and successful than the general population ... if he/she learns to handle this gift and not abuse it!

A manic's mind is often racing with ideas and thoughts, thus, they can be very productive if not to exceed the limits ... to go off the deep end, or to tackle too much at one time.

A manic depressive's condition is caused by a chemical disorder or better known as a chemical deficiency of body salt. This salt affects the actions of one's brain activity. One cannot obtain this through table salt. In fact, table salt seems to reduce this level further even if the manic is on lithium. A manic depressive's condition is without a doubt one of the easiest forms of mental disorders or illness to treat. The most common treatment of this illness is a medication called lithium taken orally on a daily basis.

Unless your doctor is overly concerned about your condition and prescribes you an excessively high dosage of lithium, you should have little or no side effects. I personally prefer and highly recommend a newer medication called lithobid, which contains the same body salt chemical compound as lithium. Lithobid is a slow time-release tablet, as opposed to the lithium capsule, and is even smaller and easier to swallow.

Both lithium and lithobid not only control manic conditions but also have been known to prevent severe depression. Often, depression will follow a "high" manic condition, where one is mentally driving the body at speeds of 200-400 m.p.h. They then become burnt-out and fall into a depression, as is the case with many manics. I personally enjoy riding my body along at 200 m.p.h. I will show you a chart later in this book and explain the cruising speeds of a manic. My body has reached speeds of 400 m.p.h., but I didn't enjoy being around myself, and I know for a fact that others didn't enjoy being around me either.

When manics are free of depression, and not too aggressive, they are not only dynamic and successful, they are often achievers, can excel, and are productive in all other facets of life. They can be easily excited yet compassionate, if they can slow themselves down long enough to do so. A manic can be profound and astonishing, as well as an outstanding individual in the community. During this "high" one is often creative with these high anxiety levels. Often, none of these great achievements can be accomplished while on too heavy doses of medication, which tends to slow this individual down. I do not encourage one to stop taking medication and encourage the manic to find a good therapist. A problem with reaching these "highs" is being able to deal with the depression that often follows an "extreme high." Believe me, this depression can be a horrible nightmare, but with proper medication and therapy, these depressions can often be prevented. I personally believe that with biofeedback, psychotherapy, and less medication, one can keep a certain "high" under control. Most manics are also daydreamers on the verge of being creative and find this impossible while on too much medication.

The title of my first book states, manic energy is a Gift from God, and many of you manics may wonder why God would give anyone such a terrible thing. Well, I could give my son a gift of a car and he could hurt or even kill himself. This is the choice one has as a manic; he can never abuse his gift. Just as my son must learn to take care of his "gift of a car" so must a manic learn to use his/her gift. Just as my son will take a drivers education course to improve his driving, so must a manic seek therapy and proper medication to use his "Gift from God" appropriately. Just remember ...God gives us the freedom to live our lives the way we choose. He doesn't control our destiny and what we do with our lives. So, don't abuse this gift.

Some of the most successful and dynamic presidents of this great nation reportedly were manics, as well as many corporate leaders. They are also in each and every other profession, as we number between 20-25 million without many even knowing they are manic. Many of us do not realize we are manic until we mentally crash — often between the age of 20 or 30. If a manic can keep it together, outstanding leadership is possible. Those who don't keep it together are in institutions and/or wasting their life away in depression.

Many young manics love to live a life of danger, thrill and excitement and enter careers that require danger and excitement. At this young age, they are often not diagnosed as manic depressive. A manic must accept responsibility and learn to face trouble with compassion and understanding instead of force, anger and self-destruction.

On the other hand, many manics are complainers, especially in a depressed state, and blame everyone else for their troubles. Their blame may be partially true, but it is not a way to recovery. If people in this condition could only tape themselves and hear themselves played back, they would more likely get this under control along with some possible psychotherapy and biofeedback as well as proper medication.

One reason a manic can be so much more productive is that he/she requires less sleep and rest. This excess energy provides them with more time to tackle the world.

Many manics, after a racing day, have difficulty getting to sleep. Many, such as myself, need medication to do so. Their minds may still be racing and they find themselves unable to relax, much less to sleep without medication. I have found that an exercise program of walking 4-6 miles a day enables me to sleep better. Others may prefer running, aerobics, bicycling, etc..

According to scientific research the average person uses only 5 percent of the brain. This is not true with a manic during his racing days, for a manic's mind is racing at high speeds. Just imagine what this world would be like if everyone increased their capabilities from one-twentieth to at least one-tenth capability. We could significantly increase our present intelligence just as many manics often do.

A manic depressive has absolutely nothing to be ashamed of. If they can deal with their highs and lows, they can be productive individuals. If only they will realize they are gifted and not abuse this gift. A manic who is in top form can run circles around a nonmanic with the same training and education. However, if one abuses this gift they will fall, only to pick themselves up again Believe me ...it's tough (often embarrassing) picking yourself up after you have fallen or crashed. Even if you don't crash, virtually no one enjoys being around a manic who seems to be racing at speeds upward to 400 m.p.h.

One frequent and important question a manic will ask is: "How can I get my family to understand me"? First, people must educate themselves and then their families. Secondly, the family must be concerned enough to educate themselves as to how to be supportive. In many cases, families think they are the victims of a mentally ill child and make no attempt to educate themselves on this subject. I can think of no one who has hurt me more than my own wife, as well as my family, since they failed to understand my behavior.

I have never been a threat to myself or society, yet have had horrifying experiences in institutions. True, I did need help, but I believe only as an outpatient, with adequate one-on-one treatment with a good therapist. Being overly talkative is no reason to institutionalize a manic. Some group therapy can also be productive in this situation. In addition to this book, there are several other good books a manic and his/her family can read on the subject. However, one should know that the better therapists are the ones you pay for instead of those usually working in state or county clinics. They are often too quick to hospitalize you. However, people should remember if they are a danger to themselves or society, they should be hospitalized.

Many manic depressives are often dysfunctional persons which means they are frequently motivated by fear. My fear is that of being locked up again. A dysfunctional person often fears being hurt by others. When a manic's behavior becomes too inappropriate, some families (as has been my case) seem to become demanding instead of understanding. When one becomes dysfunctional, he not only has fear, but often possesses defensive behavior. This describes me to a T. Defensive behavior, whether it is conscious or not, is most often based on that fear at some level.

This, along with other manic traits, can bring an awful lot of stress into a manic's family structure. If the manic is fortunate enough to have an understanding family, their family will find ways of coping and dealing with what the manic is experiencing, As in my case, I have been forced over and over to survive in dangerous institutions. However, I believe my family now understands the dangers I have experienced in these institutions. Constant appropriate therapy and institutional placement is of utmost importance. Placement where there is fighting and blood is not proper treatment for a manic, especially if he doesn't wish to fight. Nor is being institutionalized with murders, rapists and homosexuals proper treatment.

It has been my experience when in the institution to seldom see a doctor and then only for short periods of time. In addition, I can honestly say, I have been the victim of misunderstood and misinformed family. By misinformed, I mean I have had many quack doctors who have only loaded me full of drugs with little or no therapy. My family has been totally misinformed by these quacks. Believe me, I have had some good doctors and know the difference. I have no respect for a pill pusher who gives me 2 1/2 minutes of therapy and then prescribes pills to calm me down. I do not believe a psychiatrist can determine what's going on in anyone's head in 2 1/2 minutes, much less determine what medication to prescribe.

A nonviolent manic, in my opinion, should not be surrounded by violent people regardless of their problem. Clinics should be built for the nonviolent manic with qualified doctors to treat them. After all, we are looking at 20-25 million Americans alone who need this help and assistance. Some states are reported to have good clinics with very qualified doctors. However, it has been my experience that treatment facilities in North Florida, if not the entire State of Florida, are inadequate. A manic who receives inappropriate treatment is often the victim of shame, is full of anger, depression, aggression and guilt. They are often powerless since they have been committed to an institution by their own family into this possible "death-trap". I have come very close to death on several occasions while inappropriately placed in these institutions which my family thought I should be in. To avoid this, I encourage you to do some research in order to find an excellent private doctor or clinic. Remember to avoid the 2-1/2 minute "pill-pusher". Get yourself or your loved one some appropriate therapy. It is often demoralizing as well as dangerous for a manic to receive inadequate and inappropriate treatment. I believe a healthy mind requires being able to tolerate and cope with certain kinds of extremely painful feelings. If you have received improper treatment, as I have, you must put it behind you and go forward and not worry about the past.

A manic must learn to slow down, through proper therapy, biofeedback, relaxation techniques, exercise, and for religious nuturing. If you can't slow yourself down, then one day you are headed for destruction, or in my case, have already met with it and had to rebuild your life as I have. I have not totally rebuilt my life, as I long for another woman in my life who would become the new Mrs. Wessinger. My first wife was not very understanding nor did she have much knowledge about manics or how to cope and deal with one. I have changed very much, but my manic condition did cost me a family life. Regardless of the times I have been through, I have tried to be nothing less than a gentleman and a good father. However, I have been very defensive at times.

To be hypermanic is the same as being a manic, but you are going at speeds of about 200 m.p.h., as opposed to speeds up to 400 m.p.h.

Like a manic, a hypermanic is often more dynamic and successful than the general population. They are achievers. In a hypermanic condition, you have not gone as high up as a manic so you don't often crash into a deep depression. One must be careful not to become manic nor to fall into a state of depression. One must learn to read his body. I was personally hypermanic through the age of 28, as I made $143,000 my first year out of college, and was worth close to 2 million dollars by the time I was 28 and received my first manic level later, only to find out that I had given my wife a divorce settlement outrageously large. Then she fled the state against our agreement about our children, and I went immediately into a manic state due to this loss.

Manic and hypermanic people are usually individuals who possess a high anxiety level. Anxiety-ridden people are usually individuals who are quick to get intensely involved in matters that are often none of their business.

A hypermanic individual can also be hard to follow or understand, as they are often going in many different directions and often speak rapidly. They are not in a manic state but are not too far from it. Their body chemistry is the same as that of a manic, but fortunately, they have not reached high gear.

Family members and spouses are more apt to understand and deal with one in a hypermanic condition as opposed to one in a manic condition. It is most important that a hypermanic individual be on medication and receive therapy, to avoid a manic condition or even a crash, which may follow. However, one can crash without even going into a manic condition, but it is just not as likely.

A manic often has a roller-coaster career, just as I have. They often push themselves to financial ruin, only to pick up and get into high gear once again. Many dynamic and successful manics reach the top of their organization if indeed they don't end up owning it. If they are too manic, they do this often with a lack of tact, with colleagues and sabotage their advancement with destructive behavior.

A manic often makes a good-to-excellent comedian, since they are often the life of the party. Many manics are successful salespeople as well as business executives. These mild-to-moderate mood swings that manics experience, if they are not taken too far, enable them to become super-achievers.

In a society of hustlers, they are more likely to rise to the top. These mild highs are most often an asset to a manic and definitely not a liability unless one gets too manic or depressed.

A hyperverbal personality is only talkative and more friendly. The next step down would be as normal as everyone else. Any given person, not only a manic, can be hyperverbal at any given time.

Hyperverbal people should always be careful to make sure they are not dominating the conversation. If that's the case, it can often be difficult for another party to get a word in edgewise. A hyperverbal can be a great conversationalist; however, he must allow others to speak and allow them to join in the conversation.

In closing this chapter, I would like to say that I have found the drug "jegratal" quite helpful also, but I take all mine at bedtime to avoid drowsiness during the day. The main thing is you just have to trust your doctor. Education or job training for a bipolar is essential.

CHAPTER II

TYPICAL MANIC MOOD SWINGS

Howard Hughes would often spend millions on a whim for such things as a television station only to allow himself the pleasure of watching 5:00 a.m. cowboy movies. Now I ask you, is this eccentric or manic?

Howard Hughes' almost total disappearance from civilization, as well as his eccentric manic behavior and depression, suggest to us that he was a mentally ill individual in his later years. However, as we all know, he had his very productive years prior to his final years of misery.

Many manics seem to have a great desire for extramarital affairs. Since I have never had such desires, I cannot describe desires or wants these manics have. I suppose since they are so active in other aspects, of their lives, sex is no different. These "roving manics" are unfortunately often oversexed and have high-energy manic person-alities.

Ernest Hemingway and many other dynamic and creative manics killed themselves. Sylvia Plath, a dynamic novelist, did so at a time when her work was being widely acclaimed. Others, from astronauts to business tycoons, have learned to keep their gift under control and thus have continued to thrive and achieve extraordinary success.

Let us not forget the incredible manic "super woman" who rarely sleeps and constantly has high energy levels, working hours at a time, taking care of the children, as well as holding down a part-time job, or even a full-time job, as the case may be. She often gets to bed at 1:00 a.m., and if not awakened for a diaper change or sick child, is up by 6:00 a.m. and begins cleaning the house, often after only a cup of coffee, and having read the newspaper. Then she takes the kids to school, and her day actually begins. One's spouse should recognize these signs of the manic housewife, so as to avoid the ultimate "crash" they so often experience. One should help a spouse get the necessary help before disaster hits the family.

It is not uncommon for a manic individual to create an entire movie with a complete cast in a very short period of time. This is also true for artists who write, edit, and have a book ready to be published in a brief time span. It's definitely remarkable for one to create and complete such a feat or achievement. However, this is one of the "gifts" a manic has. Other such dynamic and successful people in the arts include manic producers, actors and actresses. Manic individuals, such as those just mentioned, definitely go into a manic psychosis when accomplishing these feats.

These -same individuals as well as other manics will, on occasion, usually fall into a deep depression. Some commit suicide while others stay in bed refusing to shave and shower or to take care of themselves. Believe me, this is a horrible and frightening feeling which I am glad I haven't suffered since my divorce in 1980.

Anxiety as well as depression is without a doubt easily recognized by informed friends and family members. The psychological components of anxiety are uneasiness, apprehension, verboseness, stress and tension, which show up physically in the form of a rapid heart beat, a profound perspiration, clammy hands and fidgety actions.

Twenty million Americans each year suffer from the horrible sensations of depression. Manics aren't the only ones who suffer from depression. Most of these people need help and guidance and some will refuse it. Others will commit suicide. Depression is not that difficult to treat with advanced anti-depressants and therapy.

Many milder manic conditions and hypermanic conditions are never recognized by some experts in this field. This is often because this manic is thought to be just a little dynamic and successful and nothing more than that. These same manic individuals are constantly coming up with new ideas and often successful deals, new projects to work on, and even new or additional careers that often make them wealthy. Among manics like this are the manic stockbrokers, who are, without a doubt, the sharpest, cleverest, and most energetic brokers in the firm, if indeed they don't own the firm outright themselves. These same manic stockbrokers can on occasion be totally self-destructive. They do this often when they stop taking their medication and go to mental speeds up to 400 m.p.h. They can destroy a client's portfolio in a matter of seconds when they are on a manic spending spree.

If a manic wishes to totally self-destruct, all he/she has to do is to stop taking medication, and it is bound to happen. Yes ... C-R-A-S-H, and then you must build your life back, after it has crumbled into a thousand pieces and ... that is tough to do. However, I've done it many times with the help of the Lord and my Bible by my side. During these rough days, especially, if depression is present, I highly recommend that you read the book of Job and the Proverbs. Do this from a Bible you can easily understand such as the LIVING BIBLE. Your understanding of these two books can, along with prayer, pick you up.

I even find that daily devotion gives me added strength and encouragement. Jesus once said, "I will not leave you comfortless." So let Christ walk with you. Don't walk away from him. We manics are the most productive force in America and with God on our side, along with an excellent doctor, we can remain productive and avoid the pitfalls (or at least be able to pick ourselves back up). We are leaders, and we were most likely put on this earth for this reason. Therefore, we must not abuse this Gift from God. Now let's look at the chart on the speeds of a manic depressive:

A MANIC'S SPEED CAPABILITIES
MANIC CONDITION/SPEEDS OF 400 M.P.H.

Medical Emergency! Often needs to be hospitalized if a danger to self and/or others. Otherwise extensive outpatients treatment is necessary. Extremely talkative, elated, over acting and often belligerent and incoherent. Gets very little to no sleep for days at a time. Delusional and hallucinating on occasions. Possibly violent or paranoid. Lithium medication should be carefully increased. One may need additional medication to slow down. Loves to spend money.

HYPER-MANIC CONDITION/SPEEDS OF 200 M.P.H.

Does not need hospitalization unless a threat to self and/or others. Extreme elation and excitement and very talkative. Needs and requires less sleep (4-5 hours per night). Often has many new ideas or projects to start. High energy levels and often creative. Feels on top of the world with no one capable of holding him down. Usually, there is an increased desire for sex, even someone other than a spouse. Spends and wastes money as erratically as in a manic state. Travel desires often increase, especially those with adventure and danger involved, Often dynamic and successful people, they are usually in no way destructive to self, family, or career.

HYPER-VERBAL CONDITION/SPEEDS
OF 125-150 M.P.H.

Many people (not only manics) are hyperverbal at one time or another. Often friendly and very talkative, and the life of the party. Usually very productive, successful as well as creative. Certainly a great feeling but short of feeling on top of world.

SPEEDS OF 100 M.P.H.

Just as normal as anyone who is not a manic, hypermanic or

hyperverbal individual.

SPEEDS OF 80 M.P.H.

Only a mild depression, and one most often needs only qualified professional therapy with little or no anti-depressants. A definite lack of energy. Desire for sex decreased.

SPEEDS OF 60 M.P.H.

A moderate depression is observed and should be treated with both professional therapy and anti-depressants, when considered necessary. Much less energy, noticeable decrease in appetite and sex drive, and often isolated from others. Often won't even get out of bed to shave and shower, much less go to work. Feels life is certainly not worth while, and on occasion considers suicide. Can most often be treated as an outpatient. Sleep disorder becomes serious.

SPEEDS OF 40 M.P.H.

Patient is diagnosed as suffering severe depression. Often rapid weight loss. Will often admit suicidal thoughts to others. Very withdrawn and occasionally paranoid. Some need hospitalization.

SPEEDS OF 20 M.P.H.

Diagnosed as being in extreme, severe, deep depression. Obviously suicidal, completely withdrawn and extremely agitated with those who do put up with this irrational individual. Needs hospitalization in most cases.

0 M.P.H. "THE WORST OF THE PITS"

Diagnosed as a definite medical emergency, this type of personality should be hospitalized immediately. Often unable to eat or take medication. Delusional and usually suicidal and in a stupor. Oblivious and may require tube feeding. Dangerous not to hospitalize this individual.

I have personally experienced speeds as low as 40 m.p.h. However, this was due to my last three years of marriage, as I have had no severe depression since my 1980 divorce. Speeds of 400 m.p.h. have also been experienced as my body has flown at high manic speeds. I seem to have mellowed out and settled down now.

Remember the above mentioned speeds and mentally place yourself where you have been on it. Lithium and a good psychiatrist can prevent these highs and lows without making you less productive. Lithium has been called the most wonderful drug in modern day medicine.

Some people only seek help when they are at too low a speed and neglect taking lithium so they can become manic. Believe me, no one likes to be around an out-of-control manic individual. I have found that a low dose of lithium will still allow me to be dynamic and successful and can keep me in control. Just remember, we have a God-given gift, so let's use it, not abuse it, nor let it get out of control.

CHAPTER III

THE CREATIVITY OF THE MANIC

A manic with creativity can be a fascinating individual. People around a creative manic often believe this individual is drinking or on drugs. They have, however, only cranked or pumped their brain to speeds of up to 400 m.p.h. These creative manics are flamboyant in their thought and imagination, as well as in their speech. Some misunderstood manics, including myself, have been locked up by their own families while in this creative condition. There are not enough hospital beds in this country to lock up all the creative manics. The only thing wrong with the creative manic is having a mind that creates new ideas at higher speeds than normal.

As stated earlier, a manic's body only requires four to five hours of sleep. When the mind is racing, however, one out of ten doesn't even go to sleep. Since eating is not a priority of their lives, they frequently lose weight.

Not all manic individuals are as gifted as others when it comes to creativity. Not all creative individuals are manic, but many are.

Genius and insanity have been keeping good company for at least 2,000 years and probably will continue to do so until the end of time. I have on two occasions been told by psychiatrists that I possess a very high I.Q.. When I crank or pump my brain up, I am capable of being a genius in my own areas of expertise. Needless to say, to hear this frightens me.

Sure, I've needed help at times but that is by no means the same as being insane.

Aristotle, who was associated with creativity, epilepsy, melancholia, and some depression, was eminent and successful in philosophy, politics, poetry, and the arts. He once wrote, "All have tendencies toward depression."

Until the end of the 19th century, a manic was simply referred to as an insane individual and was considered akin to a genius. During this time period, to be inspired and to be creative was simply to be mad or even insane.

In recent years a study was begun of the gifts and problems associated with creativity. Writers, for instance, reportedly have a much higher incidence of psychiatric disorders when compared with non-writers.

Manic creative individuals most often possess a lot of fear. My fear is that of being locked up again. I continue to pray that this horrible situation will never come up again.

Another school of thought maintains that creativity is simply a response to pain from such things as maladjustment. A manic 'individual who is not on too much medication is usually capable of pumping himself up into a state of creativity. The popular "Barber of Seville" was completed by Rossini in an astounding thirteen days. However, this man then fell into a deep severe depression for fourteen years and produced absolutely nothing. Later when he once again began to compose, his works were of an inferior quality. Other artists reported to have experienced extreme highs and lows include Robert Schumann, Honoré de Balzac, Ernest Hemingway and Winston Churchill.

Don't abuse this gift from God. If you or your loved ones or friends observe you getting too high, then seek some good professional help and stay on your medication.

If you abuse this gift and go to high, you only have further to fall or crash. I feel that I have crashed from the top of the world, straight through the earth and into the pits of hell. Believe me, it's horrible!

So just don't let your body and head ride too high to avoid reality, because disaster may very well follow.

Most experts agree that freeing up this neurotic conflict with proper medication and/or therapy can in fact enhance the manic's creative spirit. Manics usually attempt to receive this help after they have fallen into a severe and often deep depression when they are no longer creative at all.

CHAPTER IV

FAMOUS, DYNAMIC AND SUCCESSFUL

Abraham Lincoln

Abraham Lincoln was definitely a gifted man. He, however, suffered from recurrent periods of mental depression. These depressions were often severe during the seven years which he practiced law in Illinois and later as President of the United States. These depressions are very well documented in letters, newspapers, journals, and by all of those who personally knew him, People, not only professionals or experts in this field, often commented on his evident melancholy. Lincoln was, without a doubt, a recognized genius in his time. As has been the case with many geniuses, he suffered dearly for that honor with some horrible depressions.

Through his early twenties, Lincolns' condition seems to have been more of a hyper-manic individual and was in numerous fights. At age 29, Lincoln lost his first love, Ann Rutledge, and immediately plunged into a severe and deep depression. Most of his close friends considered him suicidal. Finally, when Lincoln did get around to seeing his physician, Dr. Anson Henry, he was told only that he had a nervous condition. As a result of his loss of a loved one, Lincoln was later described as being withdrawn, introverted, and yet, at other times, even energetic and ambitious. He was also considered one of the finest trial lawyers in Illinois. Lincoln, a promising politician, was known to be shy, self-doubing, and even diffident with women.

When Lincoln recovered from the loss of his first love, Ann Rutledge, he decided to marry Mary Tood. However, he didn't show up for the wedding, and was later found by his friends at daybreak, walking alone, desperate, restless and severely depressed. Once again, suicide became a threat, and he was believed insane by Mary Todd and several close friends. Despite her frustrating embarrassment, Mary Todd's love and devotion for Lincoln continued, which eventually resulted in their marriage, once. Lincoln gained control of himself.

Few people got to know this introverted Lincoln. Most associates, including his physician, couldn't understand what he was experiencing or feeling. Lincoln could at times pump himself up to a hypermanic condition, that would later become a manic condition. At that time, he was known to have gregarious behavior and could be the life of any party. He would tell stories, laugh, be very talkative, and adapt to any situation or environment. He could, however, turn completely around with a drastic mood swing and take himself back to a moody condition, with a secretive and fearful state of mind.

His biggest rival in Illinois or elsewhere, the story goes, was .the magnetic and popular Stephen Douglas. It was during this period that Lincoln went from a hyper-manic to a manic condition. He continued his mood swings during this period. Lincoln was, for some unknown reason, believed to be in good spirits after his crucial political defeat.

Lincoln continued to fight on and eventually won the 1860 nomination as the Republican candidate for President of the United States and was elected to the presidency.

Historical records indicate that his eighteen months as President were rather inefficient, as he was constantly fighting off depression. The worst was yet to come, however, when his son died, which was the second loss of one he loved so dearly. This was his first severe and deep depression during his Presidency.

Teddy Roosevelt

Teddy Roosevelt was the next President, some believe, to have been manic. Unlike Lincoln, Roosevelt was very competent and capable. He also had a very flamboyant personality. His unimpressive days at Harvard gave no indication that he would be such a successful politician. While attending Harvard, he had few friends and was often referred to as talkative, nervous, and a big joker. In addition, he was very depressed at Harvard.

Roosevelt married Alice Lee in 1878 who seemed to discourage his eagerness. She did save him from totally exhausting himself many times and turned out to be his salvation. Unfortunately, her life ended 4 years after their marriage while giving birth to their daughter, February 14, 1884. It was no Valentine's Day for Roosevelt, as his grieving was indeed severe. However, no serious depression, as experienced previously, occurred.

Roosevelt, apparently, was only hyper-manic during his younger years but by this time had become manic. In 1899, Roosevelt was Governor of the State of New York and appeared to be as manic as ever. After only one term, He put himself forward as a vice presidential candidate and after manic campaigning ... WON! McKinley, who was President at this time, was assassinated in September of 1901, and Roosevelt was sworn in as president at the age of 43, the youngest president ever to be in office. Roosevelt, at this time, was at his highest manic level. He would have long days, at his desk by 7:30 a.m. and working long past midnight with the little sleep required in a manic condition. When entirely too manic, he would hire a professional fighter who could, after a good fight, always knock him out.

As Governor of New York, and during his Presidency, he wrote over 150,000 letters in almost manic condition. Roosevelt retired from office in 1908 when Howard Taft, a comparative slow poke, was elected. Roosevelt remained on a high and began a trip through Europe. He had a wonderful time but, becoming very bored with retirement, decided to attempt a third term as President. Roosevelt just had absolutely no desire to retire.

Winston Churchill

Winston Churchill is believed by some to have been an alcoholic
as well as a manic depressive.

Churchill began his long career in 1906 and became Prime Minister of Britain at the time of the Second World War. His life, including
his life-long career in politics, was turbulent, since his own bizarre
and eccentric energies are believed to have done him in every time
he reached a manic state of mind.

Churchill was known to be reckless in both leadership and his
personal life. He was brilliant but undoubtedly the most hardheaded
prime minister Great Britain has ever had. On many occasions, his
peers simply thought he had totally lost his mind.

Due to a great capacity and love for his work, Churchill often
worked at his desk all night. Churchill's "Black Dog Days" and deep
depressions are certainly well known. Despite being an alcoholic, he
lived to the ripe old age of 90. He died in 1968, after ten years of
major health problems including one heart attack, two strokes and
two operations. However, to his last breath, Churchill, like many other
manics, never complained of fatigue.

Howard Hughes

Howard Hughes, executive entrepreneur, acquired his wealth from
an inheritance amounting to a reported $871,000. He wasted no time
building an empire and a fortune worth over $2 billion as a manufac-
turer of oil and tools, movie-maker, aerospace manufacturer and fin-
ancier. Hughes was often shy and withdrawn in public but could be a
tyrant around his staff as well as extremely eccentric in his business
dealings. Hughes and his manic behavior built a dynasty before he
died, but he became a lonely man in total recluse.

Ernest Hemingway

Ernest Hemingway, is widely recognized as one of the great

authors of the 20th Century. His biggest achievement was to have received the Nobel Prize for Literature in 1954.

Upon graduation in 1917, he decided to forego college and began work immediately for the KANSAS CITY STAR. At the STAR he learned much that was to be helpful in his eventual career as a writer. He wanted to fight in World War I but was rejected due to an earlier eye injury. His manic drive to be in the war resulted in his becoming an ambulance driver for the Red Cross. He was then seriously wounded in Italy and subsequently decorated for bravery by the Italians.

In the years that followed, he divorced three wives. During the Thirties he spent much of his time in Spain, Africa and Florida writing of his experiences as a sportsman and adventures as a bull fighter, big game hunter and deep sea fisherman. Hemingway became one of the most colorful and public men of his time. Subsequently, his manic energy led him to become involved as a correspondent on the loyalist side in the Spanish Civil War and with the army in World War 11. In World War II, he became a legendary figure, fighting more often than he wrote. He was then better known for his military than journalistic achievements.

He produced six novels, 50 short stories, and left much work unpublished. Among his outstanding works were *The Sun Also Rises (1926), To Have and Have Not, For Whom the Bell Tolls (1940), and The Old Man and the Sea (1952).*

Grace under pressure was Hemingway's definition of courage, a quality with which much of his life and work is concerned. He believed life was painful and complex. The only way to survive this is to face what comes with honor, dignity, strength, knowledge and endurance. These principles make up what is known as the Hemingway Code. His followers were known as Code Heroes. Hemingway's overall message, however, especially as expressed in "The Old Man and the Sea" is that, although life is a lonely, losing battle, man can dominate so that his loss has dignity and is itself a victory.

Hemingway's manic energy took a mood swing into severe and

deep depression along with loss of memory. He was hospitalized twice at the Mayo Clinic, only to take his own life with a shotgun upon his second release.

There are many others I could mention, but their families prefer not. And I have found that the giant corporate leaders alive today wish to keep it private. So, out of courtesy I grant them their wish.

One of my great uncle's President, Zachary Taylor, was most likely bipolar, along with one other President who I wont mention for the sake of his children.

CHAPTER V

THE MANIC BUSINESS EXECUTIVE
AND THE BIOLOGICAL CLOCK

Many manic businessmen and women are known as what experts call the 48-hour manic depressive business executive. For the first 24 hours, they are elated, talkative, dynamic and often driving their brain at excessive speeds, while constantly wheeling and dealing at a conference table or on the telephone. During the last 24 hours of this clock-cycle, they hide from their peers and employers and often refuse telephone calls. They stay away from any form of activity, all very much the result of the fear they are experiencing. Some just want to go to bed or hide somewhere. Many manic depressives with this 48-hour biological clock condition of mood-swings are often put on anti-depressants to avoid low days. The result in many such cases is that highs are often accentuated to the point of manic psychosis.

Many manic individuals attempt to buy off their doctor to avoid taking medication but, of course, tell their family that they are on medication. There are very few 48-hour manics that have this built-in 48-hour biological clock.

Psychiatric disorders can and often do follow the biological clock of the manic depressive individual. This often is attributed to the result of environmental changes in the atmosphere, such as that of a full ' moon madness which is the source of the word lunacy.

At the time of a full moon madness one may not even be able to get available bed space in a clinic or hospital, as they are often packed full at this time.

Women who experience this condition in their menstrual cycle usually follow a 28-day lunar clock, Approximately 60% of all women experience some kind of mood change within the cycle, especially during the four to five days before and during their menstrual period. These mood changes often result from disturbances in water and sodium retention which is related to abrupt hormonal changes during one's mid-cycle. A few women suffer premenstrual tension so severe that they become almost psychotic for several days each month.

CHAPTER VI

THE MANIC DEPRESSIVE ON ALCOHOL
AND DRUGS:
RESULTS, REACTIONS AND DANGERS

One of the most common indicators of depression for manic depressive individuals is a growing dependency on alcohol, sleeping medication, and other drugs. These drugs may promote a momentary relief from the surface anxiety and from the lack of energy which is associated with the underlying depression.

It is believed by most experts that alcohol was the first tranquilizer known to man. Alcohol is a depressant. For this reason alone, manics have no business drinking. Alcohol can also reduce the lithium level after extensive drinking.

Recent studies by experts in this field reveal that manic depression and alcoholism go hand-in-hand and may be related genetically. A manic should note that alcohol reduces the lithium level of a manic depressive and with excessive or continued use can lead one to a manic condition. This has happened to me and induced me to almost quit. A manic not on too much medication can bring about a high without alcohol.

We don't normally think of alcohol and nicotine as drugs; however, both can be as addictive as heroin, cocaine, barbiturates, and amphetomines. A depressed individual, whether manic depressive or not, is the biggest abuser of both alcohol and drugs. Most manics

feel cheated and angry if they are not prescribed some form of medication after visiting a doctor. Therefore, they will often self-prescribe
either alcohol or an illegal drug substance. Doctors write as many as
800 million prescriptions to Americans each year of which 1/4 are
for mood changing drugs, such as lithium and anti-depressants. This
is simply astonishing when you realize there are approximately 240
million Americans.

At any sign of discomfort, which can be less than a simple headache, these drug abusers reach for a pill. In many cases they get no
relief from this discomfort but only a buzz or dizzy, feeling, if the
pills are potent enough to do so.

Narcotics, opium, morphine, codeine and heroin are all derived
from the poppy plant, which has grown and cultivated by the
Sumerians as early as 5,000 B.C. European doctors have used opium
to treat a number of ailments, such as deafness, asthma, jaundice,
female troubles, as well as depression, then referred to as melancholia. This first began in the West sometime in the 1500s.

Cocaine, as dangerous as it has always been, was first promoted as
a local anesthetic. This drug does, however, have one good effect
which is to block conductions of nerve impulses.

Marijuana's first use was as early as 2737 B.C. and has had a long
and close association with man and his mood along with other dangerous, deadly, and now illegal drugs. One Chinese Medical Book
lists marijuana as a drug for the relief of symptoms of gout, rheuma-
tism, malaria, here beri, female weakness, constipation, as well as
absentmindedness. The Hindus in approximately 400 B.C. believed
it suitable for religious purposes only. In time, this drug spread
throughout the entire globe.

A total of 100 million Americans drink alcohol each year, and at
least 10 million have some form of a drinking problem. Even worse,
many of these are known to be alcoholics who often drink themselves into debt or death. Approximately half or more of the total
deaths from auto accidents involve a drunk driver.

Barbiturates and sedatives, better known as downers, are very much
like alcohol, in that they too depress the central nervous system. As

for the manic depressive who is abusing alcohol, the alcohol they are consuming often sabotages their lithium treatment. A manic depressive illness cannot be treated until alcoholism is treated.

Alcohol is a drug. When it is ingested, there are predictable effects on the body. Alcohol, unlike most foods, requires no digestion before it is absorbed. Alcohol is also useless as a food. It contains calories but has no vitamins, minerals, or other essential substances. When alcohol is present it interferes with the body's ability to use other sources of energy. Most foods, after digestion, can be stored in the body for future use. Alcohol cannot. It circulates in the blood or tissue fluids until it is disposed of by the process of oxidation.

As soon as alcohol is drunk, it enters the stomach. Twenty percent of the alcohol passes through the stomach wall into the bloodstream. Eighty percent of the alcohol passes from the stomach into the small intestine where most of the alcohol then enters the bloodstream. The bloodstream then carries the alcohol to all parts of the body, such as the brain, heart, and liver. When alcohol enters the liver it is changed into water and carbon dioxide. This process is called oxidation. The liver can only oxidize one-half ounce of alcohol an hour. This means that until the liver has time to oxidize an entire half ounce of alcohol, the rest keeps passing through other parts of the body, including the brain. One-half ounce of alcohol is the equivalent of one glass of wine (5 ounces), one can of beer (12 ounces), or one shot glass of liquor (11/2 ounces).

A very important function of the liver is the maintenance of a proper blood sugar level. Sugar is the only source of energy the brain cells can use. When alcohol is present in the system the liver focuses completely on metabolizing the alcohol. This means that it does not manufacture and release sugar into the bloodstream. The brain is then deprived of proper nourishment. Symptoms include hunger, weakness, nervousness, sweating, headache, tremor. If the level is sufficiently depressed, a coma can occur. The liver excretes 90% of alcohol in the system. Ten percent is excreted in breath, sweat and urine.

As a drug, alcohol acts as a depressant on the central nervous system. The intensity of the effect is directly related to the concentration of alcohol in the blood. The alcoholic content of the liver tissue is 64% of that in the blood; of muscle, 85%, and that of the brain 88%. Once alcohol is ingested, within two minutes the brain tissues reflect accurately the blood alcohol level. A blood alcohol level of 0.10 is sufficient in most states to be convicted of driving while intoxicated. This level represents approximately 5 drinks in one hour (2 1/2 ounces of pure alcohol). Despite alcohol's source of calories, increased exercise does not increase the speed of metabolism. Nothing will produce sobriety except time; approximately one hour for each drink.

Alcohol has different effects on different people on different occasions. Factors which influence these effects include how much one drinks, weighs, has eaten, and one's situations. Abusive drinking can lead to serious bodily damage and to an incurable disease. If you choose to drink, please do so wisely.

Lithium is commonly found in tobacco, sugarcane and seaweed. Lithium is more abundant in the earth than either lead or zinc. It is a relatively safe drug as it passes from the blood stream into the tissues and is discharged through the kidneys. Older patients often respond to lower doses as the clearance time to discharge the lithium is longer.

An extreme manic episode can be brought under control and back to normalization within one to three weeks with the use of lithium. One can take higher doses of lithium within this phase since one can tolerate more lithium during the subsequent acute manic phase. It will have to be lowered after normalization however.

One may experience tremors of the hand while on lithium. This does not mean one should discontinue its use. Caffeine may increase these tremors. I experience some tremors myself occasionally. One may need to check and get a doctor's approval to reduce the intake of lithium.

CHAPTER VII

OH, GOOD! I SEE A MANIC COMING

This chapter will deal for the most part about how to avoid being ripped off, especially, if you are a manic. Just memorize this sentence and you won't have any problem: Don't Gamble, Period!

Unless, in the past, you have proven to be a professional and successful gambler, I would still suggest that you quit while you are ahead. If it's your only successful way of making a living, then I guess you can't afford to quit.

Experts say most manics love to gamble and can't resist the temptation. Manics thoroughly enjoy the excitement of gambling. However, this manic does not enjoy it at all. Many manics cannot wait for their pay checks, only to blow them at the race track, black jack or whatever they most enjoy gambling at. The manic gets an instant high as well as a feeling of power when he is winning. However, you don't have to be manic to become a compulsive gambler.

I have spoken of the high and the power one feels from winning. Now I will write about the compulsive gambler who often does not quit until he has destroyed everything he originally loved including his family and possessions seeking the high and power one feels from winning. At this point, as the individual looks into the mirror, he often notices a very depressed individual.

The life-style of a manic at speeds of 400 m.p.h. tends to be totally wasteful to the point of spending that last quarter to get a ride home by using a pay phone. This manic will go on an extensive buying spree for the sheer joy of spending as much money as possible. One extreme example of this is a man who threw $50,000 out his window, only to call his bank for more money to waste.

These manics or hypermanics are often not out of touch with reality. The constant love of wheeling and dealing for high and powerful feelings and a constant need for money are some of the many classical manic symptoms.

The manic entrepreneur may see himself as a corporate bullfighter, wheeling and dealing with the wall Street Brokerage Houses. Identical to the manic gambler, the manic businessman certainly has an advantage over competitors, if he can drive through the deal at speeds below 300 m.p.h.

Manic businessmen and women make much more successful business executives than they do gamblers. In fact, many of the most successful business executives and entrepreneurs are manic. Believe me, there is much gambling involved in owning your own business, and it is a challenge for a manic.

Manic businessmen and women often have a definite fear of vacations, unless they are in a mild form of depression. The reason is simple; they are extremely hyperactive and find enforced leisure to be a definitive form of torture and unpleasantness. This may not be the case if one has an opportunity to sky dive, snow ski, or other dangerous and exciting activities.

After wheeling and dealing all day long, many manics often wish they had a longer day, even though their day is already as much as 4 hours longer, since a manic requires up to 4 hours less sleep than a non-manic individual.

Whether you are a manic gambler in a casino or a manic who is wheeling and dealing, or even a successful manic businessman or woman, you should have non-manic expert advisors to keep you from gambling away all you own.

If this wheeling and dealing manic gets too high, he only has further to fall and may on occasion crash into severe and deep depression when they lack a desire to go to work. You can't abuse this gift and not expect to fall apart at the seams. If a manic remains crashed for too long, the result is the loss of a business or even a job as the case may be. Like the gambler, he can lose everything. Many may commit suicide, especially in a severe and deep depression and even more often when they have lost almost all of their once successful empire. These successful people often just can't handle defeat, even though God and all of you know they can rebuild this same successful empire once again. This is exactly what I am doing at the present: rebuilding the empire that I had 8 years ago. I am beginning to see daylight once again with the help of the Lord. I have had some terrible times but have never desired to kill myself, for God has never deserted me nor have I deserted him.

I will be successful and on top of the world once again because I have this gift from God, and have to learn not to abuse it, to keep it under control. To that end, I have found that a daily devotion and some Bible reading the first thing each morning provides invaluable guidance. Without the Lord, suicide would have been much more likely for me and for many others who have made it through rough times with the help of the Lord.

CHAPTER VIII

THE DOWNSIDE OF DEPRESSION
AND
WHAT WE KNOW

Something is being done by many experts in the field of manic depressive illness for the treatment of people who are overcome by feelings of low energy and depression.

Depression which often follows one's manic state is a most horrible mental illness. It is also the common psychiatric problem for which manic depressive individuals seek help. Unfortunately, you don't have to be manic depressive to suffer from depression. If you do experience depression, I highly recommend that you read the book of Job and then Proverbs in your Bible. If you don't have a Bible that you can read and understand, then buy one such as the Living Bible.

Depression and elation are manic depressive experiences described by Old testament writers and early Greeks and Romans. During this historical period, philosophers, historians, poets, novelists and a few in the medical profession accepted mental depression as part of the human condition. Furthermore, they noted it could range from sporadic moments of misery and joy to prolonged periods of extreme despondency or elation, indicating a serious mental disorder. Such disorders or mood swings through the centuries have been misdiagnosed by many less than professional doctors. However, many manic depressive individuals who have not been led to suicide have continued to be uncontrollable during their illness, even with treatment from the best doctors in the field.

We are presently undergoing our third and most spectacular revolution in the treatment of emotional illness. Finally, in recent years, a major chemical breakthrough, lithium treatment offers prevention against manic depression or recurrent depression.

These chemically treatable mood disorders can now be easily recognized and are characterized by what most experts in the field refer to as recurrent mood swings . Most experts in the field of manic depression treat these emotional disorders with drugs to alter or correct any abnormal body chemistry. In addition, psychotherapy and biofeedback should not be ruled out. One's doctor can treat these symptoms with both medication and therapy and can usually get quicker results than with medication alone.

Before lithium came along, there was the use of straight jackets and excessive major tranquilizers used to slow the manic down and induce sleep. During this process, the side affects of retarded body movement, a mask like face with little expression, and a zombie like appearance were quite evident in these patients. I have received such treatment, and it's horrible. It has been my experience that lithium, psychotherapy and biofeedback are a much better treatment process for the patient, and recovery is much shorter. Most manic depressive patients calmed on lithium can reduce their own hyper condition. These patients are usually ready for discharge from the hospital within several weeks, if hospitalization is even necessary.

Some of these manic individuals will drive themselves too hard and will often crash after these highs into depression. One must learn to read the signs of being manic and seek professional help instead of waiting for the depression which follows. Unless one is on too much medication, he can usually remain productive and in control. If one does not seek professional help at this point, depression may set in and require commitment into a mental hospital or clinic. Outpatient treatment is less traumatizing, more practical and less expensive. A manic is often too psychotic and irrational to think about getting professional help and will ultimately crash.

Anti-depressants and shock treatment were more often used in the Sixties for serious mental depression. Today, lithium and therapy are much more prevalent. Centuries ago, treatment for a manic often involved torture and harsh treatment,

CLINICAL DEPRESSION

Clinical depression is a devastating medical disorder. It destroys people. It ravages families. It ruins careers. It affects at least one in ten Americans at some point in their lives. Yet, surprisingly and sadly, most people fail to recognize it in themselves or in their loved ones. What makes this especially tragic is that clinical depression can be treated. Mental health experts estimate that nearly 90 percent of those affected can be helped successfully.

Depression - Almost everyone knows what the word means. Or do they? In fact, the word "depression" has many different meanings. In psychiatry, depression may range from a transient, momentary feeling or emotional dejection all the way to a severe disorder that can stop a person from functioning, cause a slowdown of body processes, and even lead to death.

WHAT IS CLINICAL DEPRESSION?

The blues. The blahs. The pits. Down in the dumps. Under the weather. Lower than a snake's belly. Just about everybody has a favorite phrase to describe a depressed mood. In some ways, the condition is almost like an object; we know its location is down and its color is blue, gray, black, or sometimes no color at all. But for the most part, people regard depression as a feeling, a mood, an emotion.

WHO GETS DEPRESSED?

Depression afflicts all types of people: rich and poor, old and young, the college professor and the ditch-digger. Back to the beginning of recorded history and literature, instances of depression have been described. In the Old Testament, both King Saul and Job, from descriptions of their behavior, suffered from serious depressions. Shakespeare, too, describes instances of depression. Hamlet, the "melancholy Dane," is probably the prime example. His soliloquy on suicide, "To be or not to be," is one of the best known pieces of poetry in the English language. Novelists, poets, and dramatists throughout western history have depicted depression: Poe, Dostoevski, Hawthorne, Milton, Blake, Ibsen and Eugene O'Neill. The famous and powerful, no less than the ordinary and obscure, have endured it. Abraham Lincoln was a sufferer; Winston Churchill as well, who termed his periodic depression with chilling accuracy "the black dog." The actress Vivien Leigh, the Broadway producer Joshua Logan, responsible for such hit plays as "South Pacific," and the author Leo Tolstoy suffered some variant of the illness. More recently, Senator Thomas Eagleton and the astronaut Edwin "Buzz" Aldrin is an example that come to mind.

For some time it had been thought that depression was more common to late-middle and old age, but recent surveys indicate a higher proportion of younger persons get depressed, and that depression occurs as much or more in the 20-40 age range as in older persons. Even depression in infants, children and adolescents has been under-identified. In general, clinical depression is twice as common in women as in men. Possible reasons for this are genetic, sociocultural, hormonal, diagnostic practices, and that women seek help more often than men. All of these possibilities are receiving a great deal of research attention.

From four to ten percent of the American public now suffers from an identifiable depressive disorder. Over the course of a lifetime, perhaps 25 percent of the population will experience a major depressive episode. In fact, clinical depression is so prevalent in the United States that most people have a friend or relative who has suffered or is suffering some variant of the disorder.

CAN DEPRESSION BE TREATED?

There are a number of effective treatments available for clinical depressions; these include several specific forms of psychotherapy, a variety of anti-depressant drugs and lithium, combinations of drugs and psychotherapy, and electro-convulsive treatment (ECT). The preferred treatment depends in part on the type and severity of the depression and, in part, on factors such as the physical condition and age of the depressed person. Many people are helped by treatment, although all treatments do not work equally well for all people. Some people with recurrent unipolar or bipolar disorders have been helped substantially by long-term maintenance treatment.

WILL THE DEPRESSED PERSON RECOVER?

With adequate treatment, improvement should occur in about one month for most depressions. Most serious depressive episodes are self-limiting. Untreated, they can last for a year or more. Untreated episodes of mania and depression in bipolar disorder are likely to have a shorter duration: from several days or weeks to a few months. Most people return to their normal level of functioning after the episode, although in 20 to 25 percent of the cases, the disorder is chronic, causing considerable symptomatic and social impairment. Milder forms of clinical depression, i.e., cyclothymic and dysthymic disorders, untreated, are considered chronic. But it should be remembered that every person is different and reacts differently to the treatment.

WILL DEPRESSION RETURN?

Approximately 50 percent of those who have had a major clinical depressive episode will never have another one. For the remaining 50 percent, the course is variable: there may be a few episodes with intervals of many years of normal functioning, episodes may be more frequent, or may cluster. For some, the frequency of episodes will increase with advancing age. Most individuals who have one or more manic episodes will eventually also have a depressive episode. For these, the course is similarly variable. Adequate treatment can minimize or reduce the severity of the episode in many cases.'

HOW LIKELY IS THE POSSIBILITY OF SUICIDE?

Long-term follow-up studies of persons with serious clinical depressions not associated with other psychiatric disorders have found a suicide rate of 15 percent. A greater percentage of women attempt suicide, but a greater percentage of men successfully complete the act. An especially high suicide risk is a white man over the age of 45 who is separated, widowed or divorced, lives alone, and is unemployed or retired. A number of researchers have found that the likelihood of completed suicide in depressed people is related to hopelessness and negative expectations about the future, rather than to other symptoms. With treatment, these feelings can often be overcome.

WHAT CAUSES DEPRESSION?

There seems to be no single cause for clinical depression. Rather, there are a variety of factors, some of which have more weight in certain types of depressions than others. Among these factors are genetic predisposition, biological imbalances or abnormalities, personality characteristics, learned behavior and thought patterns, stressful life events, social and economic class, culture, age, and sex,

DOES DEPRESSION RUN IN FAMILIES?

There is strong evidence that a tendency toward both bipolar and some forms of nonbipolar disorders runs in families and has a genetic component. There is also speculation that learned behavior or persistent environmental conditions in some families may lead to clinical depression in successive generations.

CAN DEPRESSION BE PREVENTED?

In general, the onset of clinical depression cannot be prevented. The condition can, however, be identified in its early stages and treated. Recurrences can sometimes be prevented or the severity of the episodes markedly reduced. Young people at risk of clinical depression because of family history or immediate relatives (parent and/or siblings) with the disorder may be identified and treated early in their lives to prevent the recurrence of full-blown episodes.

WHERE CAN THE DEPRESSED PERSON GO FOR HELP?

The first line of diagnosis and treatment is often the family doctor or local clinic, where symptoms of depression can be evaluated to rule out the possibility of physical illness. Clinical depressive syndromes may require treatment by a qualified mental health professional. While treatment is often on an outpatient basis, sometimes in-patient treatment is necessary.

WHAT IS DEPRESSION?

Types of Depression

What distinguishes ordinary sadness, or feeling down from clinical depression? This question continues to concern clinicians and researchers. Some depressive conditions are clearly definable, while other states overlap in some ways with normal functioning.

The term depression has many meanings: a mood, a symptom, and a group of syndromes. The mood, feeling, state, or emotion is what many people think of when they use the word "depression." It is a pervasive feature of ordinary human experience: at various times, sadness, disappointment, frustration, discouragement, and allied states unavoidable aspects of life.

Depression can also be a symptom of a physical or psychiatric illness or other clinical condition. As a symptom, it can be associated with a number of psychiatric disorders, including schizophrenia, anxiety, neurosis, alcoholism, hysteria, and personality disorders. It is also associated with a variety of physical illnesses including disorders of the endocrine system and the central nervous system, viral diseases, and responses to certain drugs.

The clinical depressive syndromes are what mental health researchers mean when they speak of "clinical depression." This is a group of increasingly identifiable subtypes of depression based on specific sets of symptoms and associated factors. The current benchmark for clinical depression, compared to a normal depressed mood, depends on the intensity, severity, and duration of the symptoms. Generally (except in the case of bereavement over the death of a loved one), if the depressed mood and associated symptoms last for more than 2 weeks, and if they are of sufficient intensity to interfere with ordinary daily activities, this is considered a clinical depressive syndrome.

In 1980, The American Psychiatric Association published the third edition of its DIAGNOSTIC AND STATISTICAL MANUAL. In this book, experts in the field defined the following types of clinical depression as "most common."

Major Depression

This condition is characterized by a depressed mood, which can run from a feeling of dullness or apathy all the way to total hopelessness and deep despair. It is often accompanied by frequent crying. Anxiety is sometimes present: the person may be tense, nervous and jittery or sad and miserable. Irritability, touchiness and anger can occur. Changes in thinking also characterize this condition: slowing down of thought, inability to concentrate, difficulty with memory, indecision. Often the person believes himself or herself to be helpless, worthless, guilty. Self-blame, lowered self-esteem, and feelings of failure are common: thoughts of suicide and sometimes active plans are not uncommon.

There is usually a series of changes in somatic or body functioning. Sleep disturbances are common: there may be difficulty getting to sleep, troubled sleep with frequent wakings, or early awakening two to three hours before the usual time) with inability to go back to sleep again. For some, the problem is oversleeping. Eating problems may occur: the most characteristic pattern is loss of appetite and weight, but increased appetite and weight sometimes also occur. Energy loss, feelings of lethargy or inertia, and slowed speech and movement may also occur, although sometimes the reverse may be true and there is agitation and hyperactivity (restlessness and pacing, for instance). Other physical changes, such as alterations in bowel habits (constipation is common), dry mouth, headaches, and a variety of aches and pains are sometimes seen.

Perhaps most characteristic in depression are the general changes in behavior: there is a loss of interest in things, people, events and activities previously considered pleasurable. A diminished capacity for affection, a loss of interest in sex, and an overall loss of satisfaction with life.

In major depression, these symptoms are marked: they range from moderate to severe and seriously interfere with or actually prevent a person from leading his or her usual life. In some cases, the condition is accompanied by psychotic symptoms, such as delusion and hallucinations.

Unipolar and Single-Episode Depressive Disorder

Approximately 50 percent of those who experience a major depression have only one serious episode in their lifetime. For the others, the condition reappears, and is called unipolar disorder (meaning recurrent major depressive episodes). The course of unipolar disorder may vary: episodes may be separated by long intervals, sometimes many years, or normal functioning, they may be closer together, or may cluster. For some, episodes increase in frequency with advancing age. Symptoms of a major depressive episode usually appear over a period of days to weeks, although sometimes they are more sudden. Untreated, an episode generally lasts an average of one year.

Manic Epidose

In this condition, the mood is elevated and euthoric (the so-called high). Irritability may also be present. People in a manic state are hyperactive, and often get by on very little, sleep. They have inflated or gradiose ideas about themselves. Their speech can be pressured and rapid. Their thoughts move very quickly from one topic to another, and they are easily distractible. They often show very poor judgement and may go on wild spending sprees, invest unwisely in business, or have indiscreet sexual relationships. Energy and sociability are increased. There are sometimes psychotic symptoms such as hallucinations and delusions. The latter are often of a grandiose variety-for example when the depressed person claims a special relationship with a celebrity or well-known political figure. The symptoms, can range from moderate to severe; with moderate symptoms, a stranger may not recognize the condition as a disorder, but those who are close to the individual may see the behavior as excessive and unusual. Manic episodes usually begin suddenly, and symptoms increase over a few days. They can last for a few days to a few months; typically they are much shorter than depressive episodes.

Bipolar Disorder

Bipolar disorder (sometimes called manic-depressive illness) is characterized by episodes of mania alternating with episodes of depression. In bipolar disorder the first episode is often manic; a very small number of people have only manic episodes. Frequently an episode of one type is followed immediately by a brief episode of the other type. In general, the episodes are more frequent and shorter than those in unipolar disorder. The course over a lifetime, as with unipolar disorder, is variable.

Dysthymic Disorder

This condition is also called "depressive neurosis." It is

characterized by depressed mood (dysphoria) or loss of interest in usual pleasures and activities, accompanied by the associated symptoms of unipolar disorder but without the severity or duration found in the latter. The condition may persist or it may be intermittent, with "normal" moods that last from a few days to a few weeks. For adults, the condition must have been present for 2 years to be diagnosed as a clinical depressive syndrome. Psychotic symptoms are not present. Dysthymic disorder can be described as mild to moderate; onset is unclear and the course is chronic.

Cyclothymic Disorder

This condition is characterized by a chronic mood disturbance of at least two years' duration, involving numerous periods of depression and hypomania (mild manic symptoms). Associated symptoms will be neither as severe nor as long-lasting as in a serious manic or depressive episode. In cyclothymic disorder, the depressive and hypomanic periods may be separated by periods of normal mood lasting for months at a time; or the two types of periods may be almost simultaneous or may alternate with each other.

Depressed and hypomanic periods are characterized by "paired symptoms." For instance, feelings of inadequacy during depressed periods and inflated self-esteem during manic periods; social withdrawal and uninhibited quest for companionship: sleeping too much and decreased need for sleep. There are no psychotic symptoms, onset is usually unclear and the disorder has a chronic course.

Social and Emotional Costs of Depression

Like a stone dropped into a pond, the impact of clinical depression spreads to encompass a far wider area than just the individual involved. "No man is an island, entire of itself; Every man is a piece of the continent, a part of the main," the poet John Donne observed over 400 years ago. This is as true in the 20th century as it was in the 16th. The effects of depression are truly far-reaching; they spread not only concentrically around the depressed person into his or her environment but can also influence future generations.

Estimates have been made of the economic costs of mental illness, drug abuse, and alcoholism in the United States. These figures are not specific for clinical depression. However, current knowledge suggests that not only does depression account for a sizable portion of mental illness in this country, but in addition, a fair percentage of drug abuse and alcoholism is caused by or related to depression. In a study done for the Alcohol, Drug Abuse and Mental Health Administration (ADAMHA), the total cost of these three conditions to America in 1977 was conservatively estimated at $106 billion. To put this figure into perspective, it is close to one-sixth of the total budget for the United States Government in 1983 ($718 billion).

Whatever percentage of these costs is caused by clinical depression it is a large one. Costs include not only treatment of the illness, but also losses connected with lowered productivity, job absenteeism, and permanent withdrawal from the work force because of illness or death. In an economic contest, productive members of society include not only the man or woman who works at a job paid in dollars, but also the housewife, whose value must be calculated in terms of services; the business or company that pays to provide treatment for employees also feels the impact of clinical depression. More difficult to calculate are the present and future losses incurred by depressed youth; school problems that lead to alterations in career and job choices are one example.

Social costs are not measurable in dollars. Clinical depression can lead to a host of related problems on the emotional level such as grief and pain; on the social level, family conflict, antisocial behavior, physical illness, and death. No one has yet been able to come close to providing a measurement for these complex chains of cause and effect, although researchers are attempting to do so. Some are observing effects of clinically depressed parents on their children; others study divorce in depressed as compared to non-depressed populations. But even these more specific areas of research cannot capture the complexity of the difficulties in an individual's life as the result of a clinical depressive episode or a series of these: love lost, relationships ended, potentials never developed, roads not taken. Multiplied by millions, the cumulative result of these individual disruptions is indeed beyond measurement.

Classifying Depression

In the search to understand and treat clinical depression, observing symptoms and obtaining the individual's history is only the beginning. The ultimate goal is to identify the causes of clinical depression, which researchers now think represents a number of conditions with somewhat similar manifestations.

One of the main problems with research in the past arose from disagreement on basic classification issues. Researchers and clinicians have used a number of different systems and topologies for clinical depression, including ones based on observation, inference, theory, and the classical medical model of disease. The range of different systems used to classify depressed subjects limited the utility of much research; in addition to questions as to whether the "types" were valid, research findings were difficult and sometimes impossible to compare and correlate with each other. In 1970, the National Institute of Mental Health (NIMH) established the Collaborative Program of the Psychobiology of Depression within its Clinical Research Branch. The object of this program was to organize and stimulate the research effort into the nature and causes of clinical depression; a major concern was refinement of existing systems of classification.

Researchers are moving toward a common terminology; however, in a subject as complex as clinical depression, a great deal still remains to be learned. Many terms and distinctions used in the past are still useful in identifying certain characteristics of clinical depressions; they may strongly correlate 'With subtypes, aid in observation, or give clues about causality. A few of the more common distinctions are described below.

Psychotic/neurotic

In early research on depression, a distinction was made between clinically depressed people who were psychotic and those who were depressed without being psychotic. Some researchers considered psychotic depression a specific condition of organic origin, as contrasted to "Neutoric" depression which was milder and thought to be largely of environmental origin. Other theorists considered that psychotic and neurotic depression were not two separate conditions, but two different ends of a single continuum. Currently, neither of these theories has been proven. One difficulty with this distinction is the multiple meanings given to both psychotic and neurotic depression. The term "psychotic depression" may refer to severity, to psychotic symptoms such as delusions and hallucinations, to severe social incapacitation, and/or to somatic symptoms. The term "neurotic depression" may be used to mean the absence of any or all the major characteristics of psychosis, or the depression stemming from "neurotic conflicts" as proposed by psychoanalytic theory.

Endogenous/nonendogenous

The concept of endogeneity in clinical depression has been used over time in a number of different ways. "Endogenous" means "coming from within." Currently, the term "endogenous depression" refers to a set of symptoms involving early morning awakening, loss of appetite and weight, disturbances of the psychomotor system such as agitation and lethargy, daily variations in mood (often, more noticeable depression in the morning), severe depressed mood and lack of reaction to environmental stimulation. Many of these symptoms involve disturbance of basic bodily functions; the endogenous condition is suspected to having more direct relationship to biological factors than some other types of depression. Recent research has shown that people characterized as endogenously depressed tend to be older and more severely ill than other depressed people, have basically normal personalities before the depressive episode, and show the greatest response to anti- depressant drug treatment.

Primary/Secondary

Clinical depression can be classified as primary: that is, the depressed person has had no previous psychiatric disorder (or has only had episodes of depression or mania); or secondary: the depressed person has a pre-existing psychiatric disorder (for example, schizophrenia or alcoholism) on which a clinical depression is superimposed. This is primarily a research distinction intended to select a group of "pure" depressive subjects for a better study of causes.

The primary/secondary distinction is also used in connection with physical illness. People who develop depressions clearly caused by or associated with certain diseases, drug responses, or other physical conditions are considered to have secondary depressions.

Unipolar/bipolar

Unipoloar disorder is defined as one depressive episode or a history of only depressive episodes, or far more rarely, one manic episode or a history of only manic episodes. Bipolar disorder, in contrast, is the occurrence of both manic and depressive episodes, either separately or concurrently. There is increasing evidence that unipolar disorders and bipolar disorders represent different types of depression, with some overlap. Information from genetic, biochemical, and pharmacological studies supports this distinction.

All of the diagnostic/typological approaches described above are categorical, that is, they consider the depressive syndrome as a discrete condition, separate from other psychic conditions. Critics of categorical approaches suggest that patterns of characteristics in clinical depressions have not yet been well enough identified to justify such typologies, that they require unnecessary narrowing of focus, and that they tend to focus exclusively on symptoms and disregard other variables. As an alternative, a multi-axial system has been proposed and is currently considered the most promising way of classifying clinical depressions. The five major axes, or factors, considered are symptoms, circumstances associated with symptoms, previous duration and course of symptoms, quality of personal relationships, and level of work functions.

There has been a tendency for researchers to type according to the predominance of either biological or psychological features. While the study of distinct "types" of depression is useful for research purposes, it seems clear to researchers and clinicians that there are large numbers of depressed people who do not show a preponderance of either set of characteristics, but are mixed. Further research must seek to bridge the two sets of factors which will allow for a more comprehensive and meaningful approach to classification.

THE ORIGINS OF DEPRESSION

Why do people become clinically depressed? Why do some people become depressed while others do not? Why do women seem more vulnerable to depression than men? What is the relationship of alcoholism to depression? Is depression "in the genes," or do we learn it? These are the kinds of questions people are asking and depression researchers are attempting to answer.

Researchers are now convinced that there is no one cause; there are many, and a number of approaches must be used to investigate causes. Thus, depression investigators now use a "multifctorial model," that is, they look for the interaction of several factors that influence the occurrence of clinical depression.

What causes Depression?

The current search for causes is complex; research investigations are often limited to a specific area. Examples include epiderniological studies which examine age, sex, social class and other variables in large groups of people; biological studies which include the examination of brain functioning and the endocrine system, as well as the observation of sleep patterns, bio-rhythms and cycles of bodily activity; physical illness and nutrition; genetics; the psychological effect of drugs; the psychologies of learning and the personality; and the examination of the effect of stress and life events.

Current researchers in depression seem to resemble the blind men examining the elephant. The biologist may have hold of the tail; the social researcher may have grabbed the ear; the psychological theoretician embraced the foot; but how these parts fit together is still unclear. To carry the analogy even further, researchers suspect that as the parts connect, they will discover not just one elephant but a whole herd of different sizes, shapes and behavior. Not only are there many causes for clinical depression that interest different people, but there are a number of different depressions. No one condition, event, or factor is absolutely responsible for clinical depression; instead, a number of influences converge along what has been called a "common pathway" that produces the depressive syndrome.

Epidemiology, the large scale study of population groups, is an important aid in investigating the causes of clinical depression. With the increasing use of these categories, refinements have been made in the study of depressed people and control groups on the basis of age, sex, and other variables. Recently, researchers in depression have concentrated on three broad categories; bipolar disorder, non-bipolar depression, and depressive symptoms. The concept of risk factor is a particularly important one for epidemiology. A risk factor is a condition which increases the likelihood of a person developing a particular disorder. Those at risk for depressive symptoms and non-bipolar clinical depression include women, the young, the lower classes, the unmarried and unattached, and those who have recently experienced an interpersonal loss. In bipolar disorder, although life events such as interpersonal loss may play a similar role in onset, neither being female nor unmarried possess an increased risk for the disorder.

In addition, studies in many countries indicate that women have more depressive symptoms and more non-bipolar clinical depression than men at a 2-to-1 ratio.

Theories   about   female   hormonal   and   endocrine   system involvement have been advanced to explain the preponderance of depression in women. Hormones do affect mood, but current evidence cannot explain the magnitude of the difference of prevalence in women as compared to men.

Research indicates that depressive reactions may be linked to oral contraceptives, premenstrual distress, chromosome-linked transmission, as well as psychological theories for age, marital status, socioeconomic status, race, religion, cultural background as well as genetic transmission.

The workings of the human body have been mapped in a gross sense, but many of the finer points are still uncharted territory. Some actions and interconnections of body organs and systems are just beginning to be explored. For example, recent research indicates that the functioning of the brain is far more complex than had previously been thought; its mechanisms extremely complicated and interactive even on the molecular level. When a disorder like clinical depression occurs, it may be triggered in a number of different places in the body, perhaps in several at once. Physical malfunctions may be set off by a number of factors, outside of the body as well as within it. These interactions are complex and still unclear, and the object of intensive investigation.

Several endocrine disorders have provided models for depressison: Hypothyroidism, a disorder of low thyroid production, manifests a depressive condition characterized by lethargy. Cushsing's disease, a disorder of the adrenals, is also characterized by depression. Gonadal hormones may provide a model for hormonally associated depressions in women.

There is a complex interaction between the brain and the various glands that compose the endocrine system. Classically, research has focused on the glands and their production and distribution of hormones to various organs in the body, but increasingly, scientists studying depressison are concentrating on neurohormones and their pathways to the glands.

Psychophysiology, which includes such areas as electroencephalogram (EEG) measurements, sleep studies, and the observation of biorhythms, is a useful component in the study of clinical depression.

Problems with sleep are common in clinical depression; EEG findings, in combination with other techniques, are being used to identify subtypes of depression connected with sleep patterns.

There is a close relationship between the state of health and clinical depression. Keeping healthy in general, while no guarantee against clinical depression, may help in preventing some types of depression and certainly keeps the body in a better state to deal with the disorder.

Clinical depression can be produced by certain physical illnesses and is associated with others. Among illnesses known to cause depressison are Addison's disease; Cushsing's disease; thyroid disorders; diabetes; some neurological disorders and chronic brain syndromes related to arteriosclerosis; syphilis; multiple sclerosis; and certain vitamin deficiencies. Many illnesses are associated with depression (that is, they are not known to "cause" depression, but the two conditions are often found together): infectious diseases such as infectious hepatitis; influenza; mononucleosis; rheumatic fever; anemia; malignancies; and endocrine disturbances.

The term "personality" is used by researchers to refer to characteristic modes of behavior which may be constitutional or acquired during development. According to theorists certain personality traits or sets of traits may create a vulnerability to depression, may effect the symptoms or the course of the depressive episode, or may occur as a result of the depression. In addition, a set of personality traits may be manifestations of a genetic endowment or indicate a predisposition to clinical depression. Here, the condition is considered to be continuous, with the personality set at the "mild" end and the depressive disorder at the "serious" end. None of these theories are mutually exclusive; in fact, they are often interconnected in research.

A number of behavioral theories have been advanced to explain clinical depression. The learned helplessness theory connects depression to repeated failure to control one's environment in an advantageous way. Recurrent punishment or the absence of positive reinforcement, along with repeated attempts to control or avoid the situation, result in passivity. Some researchers think this theory may bring about certain types of depression in women, who are generally trained to be more passive than men, and often either not rewarded or punished for attempts at environmental mastery.

The learned helplessness theory was originally developed on animal models such as dogs and rats. One basic experiment involved giving dogs an electric shock. If the dogs were unable to alter or prevent this shock, they became apathetic and withdrawn and later failed to respond even when the shock became avoidable. Thus, the dogs appeared to have "learned" to be helpless. The repetition of this experiment with different types of animals has shown that the learned helplessness effect results from the animal's inability to control the shock rather than from the shock itself Neurochemical changes resulting from learned helplessness have been found to be similar to those in animal separation loss. Therapy for this condition in animals includes "unlearning" and drugs such as anti-depressants.

Self-control theory maintains that clinically depressed people have problems because they pay more attention to negative events than to positive ones, focus on immediate rather then longer term consequences of behavior, are overly hard on themselves, attribute success to outside forces and failure to their own lack, and in general, reward themselves too little and punish themselves too much. Cognitive theory, in some ways similar to self-control theory, suggests that distorted thinking can be described briefly as a view of the world as cruel, the self as deficient and unworthy, and the future as hopeless. The cognitive model suggests that this type of thinking is developed as early as childhood and leads to greater susceptibility to depression during stressful periods later in life. Cognitive distortions include logical errors, misinterpretation of events and over-generalization.

Research on cognitive deficits in clinical depression has shown that, in fact, depressed people do show interference with ordinary ways of thinking. Poor concentration, memory loss, inability to make decisions, and confused thinking are real problems connected with clinical depression, not merely deficits the depressed person is imagining because he or she feels so dismal and self-depreciation. Matter learned when a person is in a depressed or manic state may not be remembered later on.

Reinforcement theories hold that depression is connected to few positive rewards and many negative reinforcements. Another observation is that depressive behavior may elicit sympathy and attention at first, which in itself is a kind of positive reinforcement of negative behavior, but that eventually people may tire of the depressed person's attitude and complaints, leaving him or her with fewer social outlets and fewer positive rewards. Not enough positive reinforcement, or too much anxiety attached to potentially rewarding behavior may lead to a kind of downward spiraling effect. The depressed person's attempts to socialize, when not met with success, may lead to fewer attempts, less success, and less desire to make more attempts. Depressed mood has been correlated with a decrease in activities, social deficits, shorter communications, and smaller social networks.

LIFE EVENTS AND DEPRESSION

The term "life event," as used by researchers, refers to a change in a person's social circumstance that causes a disruption in the customary pattern of living and requires adaptation. A life event can be desirable (a job promotion) or undesirable (the death of a loved one). It can also be defined in a number of other ways; whether or not it can be controlled by the individual; whether it is an "entrance" type of event (such as the birth of a baby), or an "exit" (such as a divorce); anticipated or unanticipated; major or minor; involving other people or only oneself; short term or long term; recently occurring or remote. Areas that encompass life events can be roughly broken down into health, work, home and family, personal and social, and financial.

Researchers have found that certain kinds of clusters of life events can cause or trigger clinical depressions. A number of studies have shown more "exit" events, more uncontrollable events in the 6 months prior to the onset of clinical depression than in non-depressed control groups with other psychiatric disturbances.

One study showed that clinically depressed people who responded poorly to tricyclic antidepressant drug treatment were having more undesirable, health-related, and uncontrollable life events during treatment than people who responded well to the drugs.

One researcher, studying the relationship of life events to depression in women, identified four "vulnerability factors" that appeared to increase the likelihood of a depression episode in the face of a stressful life event or events. These were unemployment, three or more children under the age of fourteen at home, lack of a confiding relationship with a partner, and childhood loss of a parent through death or separation. All four of these factors are presumed to contribute to depression by rendering an individual less able to cope with stress. Research studies based on this model have not supported it as a whole, although in some investigations certain aspects of it, such as the lack of a close confident among women (but not men), have been associated with depression. It is still not clear, however, whether specific vulnerability factors cause depression or merely coincide with it.

Depression itself may also cause stressful life events to occur. For example, a woman may become depressed following a divorce. She is irritable and begins to isolate herself At first, her friends rally around her, but as months go by, her behavior alienates many of them. Her lack of sleep and inability to concentrate interfere with her work; she is eventually fired from her job. When she emerges from the depression, perhaps a year later, she has lost not only her husband, but also her job and many of her friends. Whether this kind of pattern can actually be traced in clinical depressions is an area of research speculation. Most research to date has been done on events preceding depression or life events that depression may cause. There have been no correlations found to date between various subtypes of depression and negative life events. Further, negative life events are not apparently the precipitating event, while other events are endured without being followed by a depressive episode.

PSYCHOTHERAPY

Psychotherapies involve the presence of an interested but objective person (the therapist) and the use of talking to define and resolve problems. There are many kinds of psychotherapy but only a few that are specifically aimed at treating clinical depression. There are short-term treatments whose usual duration is six months or less. They include cognitive, behavioral, interpersonal and short-term psychodynamic psychotherapy. Cognitive/Behavioral Therapy treatment focuses on the depressed person's negative or distorted thinking patterns. It is characteristic of depressed people to minimize good events and maximize bad ones, to over-generalize and to personalize. Cognitive therapy assumes that negative thought patterns lead to depressed feelings and behaviors, and that the way to change the feelings is to change the thoughts.

Behavior Therapy assumes that depressive behaviors are learned and reinforced in the environment. Behavior therapy aims at changing not only the individual's behavior but also what is called the "reinforcement field" of the environment.

Interpersonal Psychotherapy is a form of therapy that deals primarily with disturbances in functioning between the depressed person and others in his other environment. This therapy deals with the current life situation and attempts to resolve current problems.

Psychodynamic psychotherapy: Its underlying theories see depression as a symptom of a complex set of character problems stemming from the person's early childhood experiences with the parents or other close relatives. Psychodynamic psychotherapies aim to treat the "whole person" rather than only the so called "symptoms," such as depression, that are manifested at any one particular time.

Therapies attempt to change or modify the depressed person's usual methods of dealing with others.

PHARMACOTHERAPY

There are three major types of drugs used to treat effective disorders: tricyclic antidepressants, monoamine oxidize inhibitors, and lithium. Drugs are generally used for moderate to severe depressions, although in depressions which are immediately life threatening, that is, where the person is actively suicidal or extremely malnourished, ECT is often used to treat manic episodes and for maintenance treatment of bipolar disorder.

The exact way in which these drugs work is not known, although they all alter the action and distribution in brain chemicals. Triyclic antidepressants are thought to prevent neurotransmitters in the synaptic cleft from being returned to the sending neuron, thus making more of them available for transmitting electrical impulses. The MADI drugs apparently have a similar effect, achieved, it is thought, by inhibiting the action of MAD, a brain enzyme that destroys neurotransmitters. Lithium's method of action is complex; it seems not only to influence neurotransmitter action, but also to effect electrolytes and other substances and functions of the body.

The use of computers and increasingly refined techniques, including non-invasive examination of human subjects, has become more sophisticated over the past ten years, and scientists' knowledge of brain function is accelerating at a rapid pace. However, the definitive answers are still in the future, and for the present, clinicians and the public continue to use antidepressant drugs because they work. People also use aspirin and find it quite effective, although to date no one has found out exactly why it works.

FINDING HELP WHEN TO SEEK HELP: If you, a relative or friend is experiencing some or all of these symptoms, if they persist for more than two weeks, and/or if they are causing a noticeable impairment in ordinary functioning: -Sad, depressed, or "empty" mood -Loss of interest or pleasure in ordinary activities -Decrease in sexual drive -Sleep disturbances -Eating disturbances -Decreased energy, fatigue -Feelings of pessimism, guilt, worthlessness, etc. - Activity level slows down or increases -Diminished ability to think and/or concentrate

WHERE TO SEEK HELP: A good place to start is your physician's office or your local health or mental health clinic. Other possibilities include: -Community Mental Health Center -General Hospital Psychiatry Department -University or medical school -State Hospital outpatient clinic -Family service/social agency -Private clinics or facilities Referrals to individual practitioners who treat depression may be sought through: -Family physician -County Medical Society -Local chapter of:

American Psychiatric Association
American Psychological Association
National Association of Social Workers

CHAPTER IX

MY LIFE AS A MANIC

My early years were spent at our family farm of 80 acres in Greenwood, Florida. This was not enough to support our family, so my father was a teacher in nearby Malone and later a flight instructor for the United States Air Force. I had two older sisters, Sandy and Cindy. Cindy and I have always been close while Sandy and I were always distant. My mother was a full-time mom and housekeeper for the kids and always there when Dad needed her.

We were very poor and lived out in the wilderness or the "sticks" of civilization. However, I did very much enjoy living in the country. I was constantly out in the woods and helping Dad in the fields.

My parents would often argue and occasionally fight. This upset me terribly, and I would head for my favorite stump. I would sit on this stump repeatedly and ask God to make me like that big oak tree in the back yard (tall and strong) not like the cut-down tree I felt I was (helpless).

I had a tremendous fear of hearing sometimes violent arguments between my father and mother, which occasionally resulted in my father throwing whatever was near him at the time. At this time, I would immediately return to my old tree stump and pray to God.

My father was a manic depressive until his death in 1980. He was not actually a violent man, just very verbal with his frightening voice. However, I was terribly frightened of this man I called my father, and dreaded his harsh punishment with a belt.

At age five, I was amazed when my father took me to see the Blue
Angels. To see these pilots doing stunts and to know my very own
father was a pilot and taught other young men to become jet pilots
simply amazed me. What impressed me even more was that my father took me out of school for this eventful and mindboggling show
of air acrobatics.

At this early age I felt a special relationship with God. However, I
later felt he let me down when Dad told us the Air Force base was
closing down and we would soon be moving to Tallahassee, Florida.
I was soon to be in the third grade and I would often cry myself to
sleep about having to move from the farm which we had worked so
hard to keep. I felt as if I was a part of this farm. I, too, had worked
hard on it as a young child, never complaining, as I just thought of it
as my family chores.

I attended Tallahassee Schools for the third and fourth grades, only
to find out we were moving once again. This time we moved to
Marianna, Florida, a short distance from our Greenwood farm. We
had a nice home in the woods in Marianna, and I had a cocker span-
iel I loved dearly, along with a rabbit who lived outdoors with my
dog. This rabbit and dog combination amused a lot of people.

At the end of the fifth grade, we moved once again to Tallahassee.
I was most unhappy again except glad to see my friend Doug. We
had become very close during my previous 2 years in Tallahassee.

During this period of my life, we were living in a crowded apartment along with my new brother Dennis, awaiting to build our own
house. I was most unhappy here and found myself in a different school
district from Doug. Here I found a new friend in quiet and shy Charles.
We played football almost every afternoon to the point that I began
to love it, and I became quite good.

At age ten one Sunday I was in the Chapel of St. Paul's Methodist
Church, when God spoke to me or sent me a message saying, "Son,
be a minister of my Faith." It was a strong message that has lasted
through the years and was not to be my only communication with
God.

In the sixth grade, I was voted "most likely to succeed." I always did feel as though I would accomplish a lot in life and this award showed that other people believed in me too. Before I knew it, I had advanced from sixth grade elementary to seventh grade in junior high school. Doug and I were once again together in junior high school.

My father bought two beautiful acres of land overlooking Lake Jackson in Tallahassee. He and I both worked very hard to clear off the first acre so the contractor could start construction on our house. All we had to work with were axes and sling blades, but, believe me, these two manics enjoyed the hard workout. I was very proud of my father, who had never had it easy in life, and I was most happy to live in a very prestigious neighborhood once our home was built.

I met and became very dear friends with Tom and Sally Overstreet, with whom I did yard work. Later, I began to babysit for this wonderful couple and in later years was considered to be part of the family along with their two sons, Tom Jr., and Jeff, as well as their two beautiful daughters, Kelly and Kathy. I referred to Tom and Sally as my godparents. I felt more like part of the family here, as my father never had taken the time to be with me unless we were working together. He never had thrown a baseball or football to me. I had become hurt and rejected as a child, and Tom and Sally recognized this and became fantastic godparents. I would do their yard work as well as babysit. Tom and Sally provided me with my own bedroom, if I desired to stay over on nights I stayed late, even though my house was only 100 yards or less away. Dad began to resist the relationship I had with Tom who was spending a lot of time raising me. So Dad insisted that I clear off the back acre alone, as he said he was too busy to help. I did just that with only an axe and a sling blade and still kept up my godparents' yard. Tom paid well for my work. However, Dad paid me only two dollars a day.

Then I got a summer job in the construction business to pay for the biggest mistake I ever bought-a motorcycle, that would almost kill me. I remained very close to Tom and Sally, and I soon realized that Tom would be a strong male influence. I admired and still do this man who had so much love for his family and included me in the family. He would spend a lot of time with us, and he would also coach his sons' baseball and football teams. I have never seen so much love and affection in a family, and I was proud to be a part of it.

One day there was a terrible forest fire behind our house destroying maybe two hundred acres. Something, maybe God, told me not to let these beautiful damaged dogwoods die. I rounded up all the dogwoods I could save and took them to our back acre and began caring for them. Then I began to root azaleas, box woods, and others. I soon began to realize I had started my own business-to be called Wessinger Nursery.

I was thoroughly enjoying the nursery business when my father approached me, telling me I was making too big a mess on his back acre. I felt this was a very cruel thing to say, since I cleared the back acre off myself and without his help. In anger, I simply gave my nursery business to my father, telling him to run it the way he wished. I soon got a paper route instead and between this, school, yard work, and babysitting for the Overstreets, I had no time left. I told Dad I would not do any more yard work for him, as I also had to make a living. My father and I became very distant. The Overstreets both recognized I had a strong desire and needed to be loved by a father figure. Through my teenage years, Tom was to be this father figure.

The relationship with my mother was very good, as she was very loving and understanding about my relationship with my godmother, Sally Overstreet. But my father was just unable to show me the love, warmth and affection I felt from my godfather. I know my father had it rough all his life, and I later forgave him for his lack of fatherhood when we became very close in later years.

I was now in the eighth grade. My grades were average for the most part except for excellent math grades. I knew then what it was that I was to be most likely to succeed in ... football with the Dallas Cowboys. I also knew that God wanted me to be a minister of his faith. So, I told God I would be a minister of his faith but not ordained. This was about the time that I told my parents I was going out for the junior high football team. They were opposed and offered me a set of drums, if I would not play football. I turned them down, and against their will, I went out for the team making first string. I became the halfback and defensive back and the fastest man on the team. After football season, I joined the track team. I was more successful in track than in football. Soon, the last year of junior high school rolled around and I had another good year in football. Then on February, 1967, my life changed.

I was on my way from my newspaper headquarters in downtown Tallahassee and on my way to school when a horrible thing happened. I was in the left lane of a one-way street and a lady in the right lane made a left hand turn from this right lane off the one way. I went 48 feet through the air without a helmet on. I looked up and saw a church steeple, and I knew I was alive. My left shoulder, however, was shattered in four places and my neck was broken, along with a severe concussion.

It wasn't found out until years later that my neck was broken. I complained of severe pain to the attending doctor, but he only took one quick x-ray and said nothing was wrong. The lady's insurance company gave me the balance of her insurance medical bills. It was only $3,200 and dad took $1,200. He bought him a used car against my wishes and said the remaining $2,000 could be used for my education. He told me the car he bought was for his "pain and suffering." Dad was, however, at the hospital constantly when I needed him along with my mother.

Needless to say, the saddest thing was that my football career was over and there would be no Dallas Cowboys for me in this lifetime. Upon graduating from junior high that year, I was chosen "most friendly and dependable."

Upon entering high school the next year, tenth grade, I attempted to play football. However, the pain in my neck became so severe that I was forced to quit. Then I enrolled in a work release program (DCT) that allowed me to leave school for work at a local shoe store. After working at the shoe store each day, I worked evenings selling cemetery lots. My manic drive enabled me to make as much as sixty dollars an hour.

Before high school graduation, I made enough money to sell my 1962 Dodge and pay for a brand new 1970 Dodge Charger 500-SE

(Special Edition), with a magnum engine. This car was bright blue
metallic with a white vinyl top, white lettered tires and light blue
leather interior. I had without a doubt the most beautiful and fastest
car in the high school parking lot. My car would drive at speeds up to
172 m.p.h., and if the police or highway patrol got behind me, I would
often outrun them, if they weren't already close enough to get my tag
number. I would pretend that I was the famous race car driver Buddy
Baker, who at that time was driving a 1970 Dodge Charger. On these
occasions, I was very manic, only I didn't know it, much less the
definition of the word. I had a driving record that looked like the
Sears catalog.

Going to school and working two jobs was also a sign of being
hyper or manic. My close high school friends were also "go-getters"
to some extent, as they began working at an early age. I had no close
lazy friends. We all worked and supported ourselves.

I went to school only about four hours a day and I was lucky to
show up three to four days a week, as I often skipped and found that
my mother would cover for me. Instead of bringing my gym shorts
home to wash, I would bring a bathing suit home. We had started a
club called the Leon Drinker's Association (LDA), and I would spend
many a school day at our clubhouse. My godparents also gave me a
key to their beach cottage on the Gulf. Needless to say, much of my
time was spent at the beach, and I never had trouble loading my car
up with friends to go. While in high school I met and fell in love with
a tall and beautiful blonde by the name of Pam. I was later to constantly argue with her, but we loved each other very much and even
more so after we made up. It just seemed to make the love that much
stronger.

After my promising football career ended due to my injuries, I
began to drink beer and liquor heavily. I told myself that it was due
to the extreme throbbing pain from my motorcycle injuries. I would
often drink as much as seven nights a week and even during school
hours. By this time, I was sixteen years of age, and the Overstreets
allowed me to use their large pool table and recreation room. They
knew that if I wanted to drink they probably couldn't stop me, so

they allowed me to do so at their house as long as I didn't drink on the highway. A guy named Ronnie became my closest and dearest friend. In these days, we would spend almost every night together drinking and shooting pool. Other friends would come along but none so dear to me as Ronnie.

Needless to say, with my beautiful fast car, a beach cottage, club house, godparents and my house with the pool table, I was a very popular guy in high school. I was vice president of the drinking club, so that earned me my own private bedroom in the club house. At times, I wondered what kind of energy I had that allowed me to attend school, work two jobs, drink every night until midnight and get up the next morning and go full speed again. I first thought it was just will and determination, only to realize in later years that I was a very gifted man. However, at this time, I was abusing this gift with my constant drinking.

Doug and I were still friends at school but not so close. The only reason I could figure was that I was so popular, and he may have felt left out. However, Ronnie was not popular and he was my dearest and closest friend because he was always there to talk to me or help me with a problem. He was also an excellent mechanic for my "charger" and kept it S-O-U-P-E-D U-P.

Prior to graduation, I jumped on Doug one evening and cleaned his clock enough to send him to the hospital for stitches. I did this because he hurt a young lady very dear to me. However, we made up the next day. I forgave him for the horrible thing he had done and we were once again just friends. There were no awards or honors given out in high school, short of the honor society. However, if there had been, I'm sure I would have been given a couple for "most days skipped" or "most popular,"

I continued to be very close to the Overstreets and to babysit their four children. I knew very little about girls, but I taught the boys to be tough and we played ball quite often. My parents disliked and resented this relationship with the Overstreets. Up until three years before my dad's death (at which time I saved his life), he was extremely jealous of my close relationship with Tom. Don't get me wrong, my father loved me very much. However, at times in my life, I also needed for him to show me more. His near death is what apparently made him realize this, and I Praise the Lord for the new father and son relationship we found.

At this time, I spent most of my free time at the Overstreets, and would even stay over when I could get away with it. One Christmas they gave me a beautiful cue stick with the case inscribed, "Diamond Jim." From that point on the recreation room became "Diamond Jim's Pool Hall."

We opened our gifts at my parents' house and celebrated a quiet Christmas Eve. However, bright and early Christmas day, I hurried next door for a Christmas that seemed filled with much more love, warmth, and affection between all of us as if I were really part of the family.

No one ever called me Jim anymore as all my friends began to call me Diamond or Diamond Jim.

I was soon to say good-bye to high school and would be on my way to college. One of the wonderful memories I left behind was that of Pam. I love this lady now more than ever.

During this time in my life, my father had become very successful. He was Director of Administration for all the mental retardation centers in the state. He later became budget director for the entire Health and Rehabilitative Services-Division with 36,000 employees. I was pleased to have my father tell me that he was proud of my plans to attend college. He agreed to help me but did expect me to "pull my own weight." I was very happy to hear this, as I knew I couldn't continue to support myself and afford college without working day and night. Also my dear grandmother helped me out a little each Christmas, and I was most thankful for her concern for my future.

Prior to entering college, I received my draft notice, probably for Vietnam. As dangerous as it would be, I was in no way opposed to serving my country or facing death. I didn't know that I was later to be diagnosed as manic, but it was this drive that actually gave me an urge to go to war on behalf of peace and democracy. At the

Jacksonville Inductee Center, they began to "light into me" about my injuries and the medication I was taking along with the pain I was experiencing. In return, I said, "Look here, you little S.O.B., I'll whip your ass and clean your clock if you as much as call me a liar again." I was in no way trying to get out of being drafted. I was only telling the truth to his questions. The little shrimp of a man shut up before I jumped on him and quickly wrote some kind of a coded message on my papers which I could not read or understand until later.

Due to the nerve damage I had in my ears from my motorcycle wreck, I failed the hearing test only to have them pass me anyway. I also flunked the eye test, but passed as well. I soon understood what the coded message meant. . . "Pass the S.O.B. regardless of his health." At the end of the center's line was a medical director who told an old high school friend of mine that he was rejected because of his flat feet. There I stood next in line and the first thing he said was, "You must have made the sergeant mad as hell at you for some reason." I told him I didn't like the sergeant's manners. Since he was indeed the medical director in charge of this facility, he was not going to issue me a bus ticket to basic training but instead put me in for tests at the U.S. Naval Hospital in Jacksonville for a couple of days.

After extensive testing and many x-rays, a surgeon gave me the bad news. He asked me how I felt about joining the service. I replied that I would be most happy to. The surgeon then looked directly at me and said, "Son, if you want to join the Navy, Army, Air Force, Marines, or even the Coast Guard for as much as a desk job, we cannot accept you as medically fit." He then informed me that my neck was broken at the fifth vertebra and that surgery was inevitable for the future. I then pleaded with this surgeon that if he and his hospital could repair and relieve the terrible pain in my neck, I would serve my country any way they saw fit. Needless to say, this doctor refused to grant my request and said that it would most likely be impossible ever to relieve the severe pain I was experiencing in my neck. I thanked the doctor for the time he spent with me and was immediately transported back to Tallahassee.

Upon my return to Tallahassee I found a neurosurgeon that gave me a 50/50 chance of ever getting up or even walking again after surgery. Extremely frightened and frustrated, I left this physician's office never to return. I became extremely depressed and started feeling very sorry for myself. I managed to put this all behind me as the horrible summer ended. I returned to my thoughts of college. I became grateful for Dad's promise to help me financially with college. He was beginning to show he was proud of me, and I began to stay home more to study.

I decided to follow my dad's footsteps in accounting. After completing community college, I entered Florida State University which I found to be very tough, I was amazed to see the dropouts in my accounting classes. My tax law professor inspired me the most. He stated that over half of his class would either drop out or fail. Not only was he tough, he was good and he assured us that passing accounting guaranteed success.

My relationship to Pam was still strong during my early college days, but due to my heavy studying, we didn't have much quality, time together. I always seemed to be studying accounting.

I made a tough decision to stop working at the shoe store and left for a better paying job (which provided me with more interesting opportunities) at a local department store. I worked in the shoe department and later became a model for men's clothing. I modeled for women's clubs and society groups, and loved it ... because they would literally buy the suits right off my back, asking if the suit would look as good on their husband as it did on me. I was also used in TV and movie commercials.

After two years of modeling and selling shoes, I felt it was time for another change. I then found employment as a counselor in a new prison in a nearby town in Florida. In a very short period of time (with my manic drive), I became the shift officer in charge of the entire facility in the absence of the chief. The chief allowed me to work the graveyard shift (midnight - 8:00 a.m.) since I was going to school. In dealing with prisoners in close security, I found it best to use my God-given talent of being manic.

Pam and I became engaged one Christmas, but it didn't last very long due to a difference in our religious beliefs and our views on raising children. Naturally, I was very hurt when she returned the engagement ring, but nevertheless wasted little time calling on one of the beautiful young women I had met earlier while working at the clothing store. Her name was Barbara.

Barbara was almost eighteen when we met for the first time, and she immediately had a crush on me. I guess you could say I was infatuated with this beautiful young lady. On our first date we watched the movie "Love Story," and I was falling in love on the rebound from Pam. We dated for about eight months before we married on June 23, 1973, for all the wrong reasons. Barbara was the daughter of a wealthy restaurant owner. I have always felt like a self-made man myself (with the help of the Lord and this God-given talent of being manic), and I was soon to resent my father-in-law. In the first place, I didn't particularly enjoy marrying into a wealthy family. Prior to the wedding date, he tried buying Barbara and me a house, and later a new Cadillac and other gifts. I immediately told him that I didn't want his money, as I knew there would be strings attached.

I was twenty-one and Barbara was 18 when we got married and bought our first house without the help of her father. It was a three-bedroom in a nice neighborhood, and with my experience in the nursery business, the yard became the most nicely landscaped yard in the neighborhood.

Well, my father-in-law started in on me again after our marriage, telling me I could come into his corporation of steak houses and to name my own price. I again refused and simply told my wife, "Everyone gets mad at their boss, and on occasion goes home cussing him, and I'm sure I would be no different even though this boss would be her father." I, personally, couldn't work for any relative for this reason. However, later my father-in-law had a good business proposal for us. He offered us a $4,000 down payment on a franchise for a steak house as a wedding gift and said we could build our own steak house. I seriously thought about it for a week and said yes, not ever dreaming that this would be a mistake.

With my father-in-law's help, I soon decided on a location in Lagrange, a small Georgia town of 26,000. 1 then realized that I had five old houses to tear down before construction was started in March, 1976, and was completed July 19, 1976. 1 had all of my employees hired by July 15 in the smallest town to ever see a Western Sizzlin'. I made $26,000 the first month. I bought Barbara a new Lincoln Continental after the first month of operation. According to my accountant and the IRS, I made $142,840 my first year. However, the more I made, the more Barbara spent. I, too, had acquired expensive taste and I allowed Barbara to talk me into bigger diamonds, jewelry, sapphires, automobiles, and more expensive clothes and home furnishings.

I was soon to find out just what kind of wife I really did marry or what she had changed into, as the case might be. We began to argue over most of the things we had agreed on before our marriage. She changed her mind about enjoying my cigars, horseback riding, boating, and every other thing I thought we shared. When I asked her why she had lied to me so much prior to our marriage she replied, "I was afraid if I didn't lie to you, you wouldn't have married me." At this point, I was even more angry and began to feel our marriage falling apart. With all this anger built up in me, I immediately went into a hypermanic state of mind.

I had hoped that our first child, soon to be born, would help our marriage. So I decided, after my daughter was born and things seemed back to normal, that I would build another steak house, partially, to protect myself in the event of a costly divorce.

At this point, the best thing in my life had happened. My first child was born on August 16, 1977, the exact day Elvis Presley died. She cried constantly until I held her, at which time she became silent and I think even grinned at me. A call to my father-in-law ended in frustration and anger when he said, "You must not have what it takes to make boys." In order to inform the public of my first child's arrival, I called my store manager and immediately heard, "The King is Dead." Being in another world at this time, I had no idea what he was talking about, and I simply said, "Well, put on the marquee at the steak house

'The Queen is Born,'" only to find out about Elvis later. As I walked out of the hospital on the day my beautiful daughter was born, I spoke to the Lord and said, "You light up my life." As I cranked the car, Debbie Boone's "You Light Up My Life" played on the radio as I said, "Thank you, Lord" again. This will always be my and my daughter's song.

I spent a lot of quality hours with my daughter Stacy, despite the long hours one must put into the restaurant business to be successful. Needless to say, her first words were Da-Da. Our marriage improved somewhat with the new addition to the family.

In June of the following summer, I took Barbara on a cruise to the Bahamas in an attempt to rekindle and save our marriage. Seven months. Later, on January 22, my son Jason Garrett was born. I was really proud now to be the father of a beautiful daughter and a hand-some son. Upon returning from the cruise, however, I realized that I was not happy with our marriage and I became somewhat manic. I bought two more franchises and soon began construction on another.

Valley, Alabama was an even smaller community than LaGrange. It was not even on the map at the time. A week before opening day of that franchise, the carpet and restaurant equipment was being installed. I had to stay at the restaurant site the entire day to check on every piece of the equipment which was worth well over $110,000. The next day everyone's eyes were burning and some employees called in sick due to extreme pain, discomfort and blurred vision. This was due to an extreme amount of carpet lint in the air from installing the carpet. I was wearing contact lenses at the time and became tempo-rarily blind and in severe pain. According to the opthalmologist, the carpet lint got behind my eyes and because of the friction the lint apparently cut my eyes as if a razor blade would have done. I prayed for five days like I had never prayed before, and woke up on the sixth day saying, "Thank you Lord," when my eyesight returned. At this point my vision became even better, and I didn't even need my con-tacts. I was later to find that I could even pass my driver's test with-out them. However, I did work while I was blind as much as I could, since the new steak house was costing me a mint everyday it was not open. What was so funny was that I got my eyesight back on April Fool's Day. However, at the time, I had no idea what the date was since I hadn't seen a newspaper or television in six days.

I simply flew down to the new steak house with every intention of opening it that evening. Then someone told me an April Fool's joke, and I said, "Oh no, it can't be April Fools." I told everyone it was my wife's birthday and immediately headed for the LaGrange Cadillac showroom where I bought her a new automobile. I took the new cadillac home and returned to the new steak house to manage the 5:00 p.m. Grand Opening. My in-laws attended the Grand Opening. My father-in-law is often rude by needlessly jumping on his employees, and he proceeded to do so with mine. I hit the roof with anger which would later prove costly to our relationship.

It was a record-breaking opening, and I made $34,000 between my two steak houses that month. Needless to say, I was certainly pleased and overjoyed and felt well blessed by the Lord.

However, with all this pressure, along with very little sleep, I became manic and knew I needed a good vacation to bring me down. So, I came home one evening and told my wife I would take her anywhere in the world she wanted to go ... if she would go. I reminded her how hard and long I had worked and that I desperately needed this test and vacation. She immediately snapped back saying she refused to go, regardless of how badly I needed the rest and relaxation. So I told her that some other boaters and I (men only) would cruise our boats from Columbus, Georgia, to Panama City Beach. I told her I would give her my daily itinerary and call her each night. She knew I had been wanting to cruise this river for sometime. She immediately informed me that she had contacted a tough lawyer, and I was told that if I took this trip, she would file for desertion of the family and throw my --- in the carport and change the door locks.

My father-in-law had not forgotten our little run-in at my last opening in the Valley Steak House. He had always promised to never crowd or hurt me by building a steak house anywhere near the ones I owned. But I soon found out by accident that he was about to open one up nearby. He specifically told me he would never build there but later wished he hadn't, since my business remained strong. He did everything but fall on his face, until he finally sold it.

For sometime I had been involved in worthwhile and rewarding activities to take my mind off of my rotten marriage. I was on the Board of Directors of the second largest church in the state of Georgia, and I spent much time and sponsored a 12-year-old child from the Big Brothers' organization. I also spent much time and money sponsoring both young boys' baseball and football teams for a couple of years. We would often meet at one of the steak houses for dinner after some of the games. I enjoyed these activities, especially the quality time I spent with these young boys. By this time, I was considered by many to be a "hell of a nice man and a pillar of the community," and was soon to be considered as a prime candidate by some politicians and prominent citizens for the next US Senate election. I was flattered but stopped such a move immediately, since I could make more money being an entrepreneur to support my wife's expensive life style.

After I realized that my marriage was totally on the rocks, I began to feel like a loser, because I had always wanted a happy marriage and a family for a lifetime. So, from the hurt and pain, I fell into a terrible depression, not even getting out of bed to check on my restaurants. My doctor was four hours away and was of little help. If a critical situation should arise at one of the restaurants, I was always there, but I just could not handle my day-to-day misery. One day, when I received two bad looking profit-and-loss statements, I snapped out of it, knowing I had to pump myself up and get into high gear. I threw away the medication and went to work.

I was not quite manic, but I was ready to build a third restaurant. I soon purchased a very good site, again in a small community and had started on the plans in something of a manic but harmless condition. Barbara decided to make a dangerous move for me. She immediately called my mother and asked her to visit. Between the two of them, they demanded that I check into a hospital in Columbus, Georgia, for treatment. Barbara was on the telephone making all the arrangements while I was out working. When I came home, she was ready to give me a pill that the doctor had prescribed. When I asked her what it was, she simply said, "I don't know, but the doctor said to take it." I was already on Lithium and sleeping pills and my body had always rejected further medication. Within five minutes of swallowing the pill, I fell out of my recliner onto the floor in front of Barbara. At this time, my mother happened to walk in and was horrified, to say the least. Since the hospital was close, Mother demanded that Barbara get me to the emergency room while Mother kept the kids. While Mom, Barbara and my sheer will power were getting me into the car, I felt I would never make it to the hospital.

Upon arriving at the emergency room, I was put on a stretcher, administered oxygen and given some kind of shot. Within minutes, I felt much better. The doctor at the emergency room immediately turned to Barbara and asked just what she had given me. She put her head down and said, "Gee, I don't know. I didn't bring the prescription bottle with me."

Upon returning to the house, Barbara and Mother both insisted that I check into the Bradley Center the next day. Unfortunately, I agreed and immediately found out that this was a mistake. In addition, I learned that the medication Barbara had given me was Haldol.

The next day I was admitted to the center, because Barbara said this was the only way to save our marriage. The doctor met me only briefly but did hear my angry statement about what he had given me the evening before. He said it was an unfortunate and terrible accident, and it would never happen again. After our short meeting, the doctor checked me into this clinic, which was soon to become a disaster for me.

I was called up for medication and looked at a certain pill, only to tell the nurse that the medication looked like Haldol, which was what I had taken the night before. She assured me it wasn't, so I swallowed it. I collapsed on the floor in pain and was unable to breathe again. The nurse simply looked over at me and then slowly walked away. Less than ten minutes before, I had been told that a young man had recently died in this clinic. I figured that I would be this week's casualty. I held on for about another five minutes, while other patients screamed for help. The nurse just sat back down behind the nurse's station.

Then a young black man came up with his mop bucket and seemed concerned and caring about my life. He told me to hold on and returned with an oxygen tank, then left again telling the nurse to get off her butt. The two came back and gave me a shot. Once again, I felt alive and out of danger. I sincerely thanked this nice young man who later told me he was in nursing school and hoped to become a doctor one day. I was angry at this nurse, who simply told me all the doctors were in a conference and there were no RNs available. She was baffled and had no idea what to do.

The next morning, I stormed to the front office and down to the resident doctor's office who was also the Medical Director of this clinic. I first asked him if he was trying to kill me. I demanded to see his PDR Book (Physician's Desk Reference) to tell me just what and how dangerous this Haldol was. He told me that it was for doctors' use only. He explained to me that the nurse had failed to see the change in medication for me, and it was a horrible mistake. Needless to say, I became very untrustworthy of this doctor. I was very upset, to say the least. I immediately returned to the ward and enrolled in each and every therapy class I could, so I could get out of this place! I spent my leisure time at the pool and playing tennis. I had several Bibles that I would read at home, but I wanted a Bible I could understand. I bought the Living Bible which I read extensively each day.

After several weeks, the resident doctor said I really didn't belong in a place like this and suggested marriage counseling with my wife to end my problems. Barbara was reluctant to come to counseling sessions but did attend. After quite a few sessions with our counselor and the doctor at the hospital, I was released. He told me he could see no reason why she couldn't change some of her attitudes toward me, as well as accept me as a hyper or simply energetic and creative husband. He also said he was impressed with my financial success. The marriage counselor's report stated that I was prepared to pick up the pieces and repair our marriage, but he was unsure about Barbara's feelings or desire to save the marriage.

The hospital physician gave me a "well ticket," and I immediately returned to LaGrange, only to find our marriage was completely destroyed and devastated as well.

I soon bought my own PDR book and learned that the Haldol Barbara and the hospital doctor had given me was indeed dangerous. In fact, heavy doses of Lithium and Haldol are quite often fatal.

I soon started going out with a good male friend, Richard, one night a week just to release the tension from my marriage. Since I was a pillar of the community we would go to either Columbus or Atlanta to avoid the local advertisement that my marriage was on the rocks. However, on none of these nights out or any other time during our marriage was I unfaithful to my wife. Richard and I continued our night out once a week for about three months. Then, I came in about 2:00 a.m. one Saturday morning and Barbara immediately said, "Let's go talk." She took me to the formal living room, which I hated and had never sat in before. She stated that I could see the children when I wanted and we would date and work on our marriage. I had known for some time that our marriage was shot, so I said, "Let's just get a divorce."

I felt relieved and later that morning, I took 12-year-old Jerry horseback riding. After spending the day with Jerry, I was reminded how much I loved kids, especially mine and could in no way part with them. I came home to ask Barbara if she would reconsider putting her offer back on the table, since I knew I wanted to see my children on a daily basis. She immediately refused but did say she would stay in LaGrange, if I would meet her terms in the divorce settlement, and allow me to see the children as often as I would like.

I immediately rented a two-bedroom townhouse and came home late each evening to an empty house to find that my kids weren't at the door yelling "Da-Da" over and over, until I picked them up and gave them a hug. Even worse, at night I would go to the closet to hang my coat up and the kids' toys would fall out reminding me even more of how much I missed them. As much as I had been through and as tough as I am, I would often cry like a baby at night. I later moved the toys in my daughter's room which I kept closed to avoid the pain, unless my kids were visiting with me.

I soon found definite evidence that my phone was being tapped. I was working long and hard hours to keep myself occupied and my mind away from the upcoming divorce. I would spend equal time between the two steak houses and my headquarters. I continued using my boat extensively as it made me feel very peaceful and relaxed flying across the top of the water skiing. My children also thoroughly enjoyed the boat. I always felt the Lord's presence while boating on the beautiful waters of West Point Lake and in the experience of sunsets on the lake.

I was soon to meet with Barbara to discuss an "out-of-court" settlement to avoid the anguish and publicity of a divorce court. We met on our patio while the babysitter kept the children. At that time, Barbara informed me that she wanted "only half of everything." Furthermore, she told me just what items and property she did demand, which was everything I had equity in. I was to be left with my old pick-up truck and one steak house of which the bank owned 98%. Of course, I could keep my boat since I owed the bank more on it than it was worth.

Needless to say, I gulped and even felt heart pains. She promised me that she would stay in the house with the children and allow me to see them anytime I desired. I soon left heartbroken over the thought of giving away the financial empire I had built and worked so hard for. However, I could only think of my two children, and I knew she would return with them to Tallahassee where her parents lived, if I didn't give her everything she wanted.

I soon found an excellent lawyer, and he and my accountant told me this would be the largest divorce settlement in northern Georgia. The LaGrange Steak House, other property, and her automobile had a net worth of about $665,000. This was not the bad news. As mentioned earlier, I had made as much as $143,000 a year in the LaGrange Steak House which had dropped somewhat now, but I still would miss at least $120,000 a year in this lost income. Against all expert advice, I decided to meet Barbara's demands so I could continue seeing my children more often. In addition to the stress of a divorce, at this time I received a most distressing call from my mother. She told me dad had cancer in four major organs and had only a few months to live. This really hurt, because Dad and I had become so close the past three years. He had become so proud of me and my accomplishments, and we had even begun to play tennis together. We had in the last three years spent much quality time together.

My father's illness and ultimate death couldn't have come at a worse time. I just felt the world was caving in on me. Needless to say, somehow I found ample time to spend with my father prior to his death. When he first became ill, I was already putting in eighteen hours a day between the two restaurants, the divorce attorney, and my office. I would often end my working day at 3:00 a.m., get into my truck and drive to Dad's bedside by 7:00 a.m. I knew that I would get very little sleep until the Lord got me through this tragedy.

My lawyer had drawn up an out-of-court settlement and made me come in to study it before deciding on such a costly move. Upon reading this settlement, all I could think of was how much I missed my children, and I broke down in tears and asked the lawyer for a Bible. After reading several passages, I skimmed over the agreement and said, "She can have it all! I just want to see my children. I can build more steak houses." I agreed to the out-of-court settlement meeting all of Barbara's demands. Two weeks later, when I called Barbara to pick up the children for a visit, I got a recording that the phone had been disconnected. Upon investigation, I learned that all of the furniture had been moved out of the house. Barbara and the children were nowhere to be found, and there was a "For Sale" sign in the yard of the house we lived in. I was devastated and at a total loss. I felt completely empty, especially since Barbara had promised to stay in LaGrange if I gave her everything. At that time, I became extremely angry and manic, for she had taken away from me the two people I loved the most. After locating Barbara and the children in Tallahassee, Barbara petitioned the court for $2,000 a month child support. Needless to say, I became more manic.

Late one evening, I was driving on the backwater of the beautiful West Point Lake noticing a full moon and clear skies. Something seemed to tell me to park my truck alongside the water. I began to look at the moon and received this overpowering message saying, "Son, your dad will die in exactly two weeks." I definitely felt the presence of the Almighty. When two weeks slowly rolled around, I was packed and ready to be at my dad's bedside once again, possibly for the last time (according to God's message). My attorney phoned just prior to my departure, telling me he and my C.P.A. had to see me immediately. I went to my attorney's office only to find the two of them wanting more financial information for the child support hearing. They were asking me to stay up almost all night to get together for them facts and figures needed for the upcoming hearing. I told these two that I couldn't get this information now, as God had told me dad was going to die tonight. They gazed at me in total amazement and shock but insisted on the importance of these facts and figures. So I agreed.

I then drove as fast as I could to my dad's bedside. As I turned my automobile into the driveway I knew I was too late. My dad had died earlier that night just as God had told me he would.

The funeral was a couple days off. Before I could even get my father buried, I received an urgent phone call from my attorney. He had called to inform me that the court date for the child support settlement had suddenly been moved up by Barbara's attorney. Thus they hit me when I was down after my father's death.

A few days after my dad's funeral, I found it necessary to return to LaGrange. It was late afternoon when I visited my attorney's office. After a visit with my attorney, I proceeded to check on my LaGrange restaurant and then on ton the Valley, Alabama, restaurant. I left the parking lot late that evening, only to notice after many turns that I was being followed. When I arrived at my headquarters in LaGrange, I quickly pulled in and got my big .357 Magnum, and set it on the seat. The man following me pulled over in a nearby gas station and resumed following me as I drove once again. Thus, I became angry and manic and decided to make this a high speed chase which lasted for several miles through downtown LaGrange. While driving with my lights off, I managed to sneak up behind him with my bright lights on, after he made the mistake of turning down a dead end street, where I cornered him. I got out of my truck pointing my .357 Magnum at him saying, "You better tell my father-in-law you quit, or I'll blow your brains out!"

I drove off wondering just what this man's intentions were. Needless to say, my lawyer was amused but happy that I was safe.

Within two days, I received an anonymous phone call from a lady, stating that a so-called hit man was in town with a $25,000 contract on my head. Upon phoning my attorney, he advised me to lay low until after my upcoming hearing. I could only hope that she believed me. My sister Sandy was soon to haunt me even worse. My mother insisted that I needed her expert bookkeeping experience for a while. I reluctantly agreed.

In the few days, several of my Valley, Alabama employees' automobiles were mysteriously damaged with slashed tires and broken windows. According to my attorney, there was still no sound evidence pointing to a guilty party so it would be worthless to even bring it up in the hearing only two days away.

On the day of the hearing (July 26, 1980), my mother and I drove to my attorney's office to meet with both my attorney and C.P.A. prior to my child support hearing. It was a short walk to the Judge's chambers where everyone was awaiting our arrival.

Barbara first took the witness stand with her attorney. I had taken my Bible and placed it directly in front of me for guidance and support. As Barbara began to speak, I pushed the Bible towards her, which seemed to make her extremely nervous. She soon got to her $2,000 a month request for child support for the two children. The judge, to my relief and surprise, began to go over the generous out-of-court settlement. He said, "Mrs. Wessinger, you are receiving the LaGrange Steak House with both considerable equity and income, and Mr. Wessinger is receiving the newly franchised Valley, Alabama Steak House. Is that correct? Then he went on to say, "Mrs. Wessinger, you are receiving this rather large house and newly acquired lake property, and Mr. Wessinger has a rented townhouse. Is that correct?" The judge kept going down this settlement and the case seemed to be going my way.

Barbara's attorney seemed very nervous and continuously pulled up one or both of his socks. As he reached into his pocket, I said, "I hope you are reaching for a pen because you already have two cigarettes lit." The judge just rolled with laughter.

It was my turn to take the witness stand. I took with me many documents including a briefcase of financial statements and seven years of tax returns. Barbara's attorney was soon standing in front of me firing tough financial questions about my earnings and worth. For each question he asked, I was able to produce documented evidence in my briefcase to support my answer. My C.P.A. made it quite clear that $2,000 a month in child support was out of my league after such a large out-of-court settlement.

We remained in the courtroom for approximately two hours before the judge dismissed us. At that time he said that it would take him four or five days to digest all of this before he ruled. Barbara and her attorney left immediately, but we stayed to have a conversation with the judge. The judge said he didn't know how much I was paying my attorney but that I had done quite well on my own. I gathered from this that the ruling would be in my favor. I laughed and thanked him at the same time, only to be shocked when I received my attorney's fee which included my C.P.A.'s time for a total cost of $17,000. I had only wished that my attorney had put in writing Barbara's and my agreement for her to remain in LaGrange with no child support.

In the meantime, we were hoping for a ruling of around $400, due to the generous out-of-court settlement. On August 1, my attorney phoned me at my office telling me that the judge had ruled on $600 a month in child support. Barbara's attorney had also petitioned the court to have me pay her attorney's fees, which was denied.

My sister Sandy was still coming up several days a week to assist me in my business affairs. I was still wondering what her motives were, since she had never seemed to me to care for my welfare before.

I was indeed manic (but harmless) after going through so much, but Sandy had convinced my mother that I should be hospitalized. Eventually, they convinced me to commit myself to the West Georgia Hospital.

In addition, my family enlisted my friend Richard into admitting me into this hospital. Before I saw the doctor, he first saw Mother, Richard and Sandy, then me with my Bible in my hand. I was glad to learn the doctor was a Christian. After thirty minutes or so of conversation with the doctor, he said that there was absolutely no medical reason for my hospitalization and that I should slow down, but return home to LaGrange immediately. I told him that I couldn't go home because both my mother and sister were in my crowded townhouse and were driving me nuts. Against his wishes, he allowed me to stay.

In the next two days, I would undergo the most thorough and complete testing I had ever undergone, including extensive x-rays, brain scans, and mental testing. Later the doctor confirmed that I had definitely been under an amount of pressure that could make anyone manic. However, away from my family I appeared to be quite normal and could probably get by without Lithium. The doctor said, however, that he would keep me on Lithium as a safety precaution. He further said that I was an extremely bright and gifted young man who did not belong in an institution, and he intended to keep me here only three more days.

Upon entering the hospital, I had given my sister, Sandy, power of attorney to run the restaurant and sign checks. I later considered this one of the biggest mistakes of my life.

Every patient including most of the staff seemed to love the way I gave spiritual strength to these patients, often healing them in a few short days. Many patients were constantly following me around and several of them referred to me as Christ who had returned to earth. Needless to say, I told them I was only one of his many messengers. One day, a very disturbed patient approached me and said very angrily, "You are not Christ, I am!

And one of us will definitely die before nightfall." He continued this outrage until he was taken away by the staff.

I called to be picked up when my five days were up. Fortunately, my mother had returned to Tallahassee, and Sandy was staying with my dear friend, Richard, as they had seemed to become somewhat fond of each other. My mother and Sandy seemed amazed and later angry that I was discharged so soon.

At this time, my sister approached me about hiring her on a full-time basis. She assured me that she wanted to own no part of the restaurant or any future restaurants that I had hoped to build. She expressed a great desire to get out of Tallahassee, after recently going through her second divorce there. I reluctantly said yes and gave her a generous salary. I had decided to take four or five days off to rest and slow down, as my doctor had prescribed.

Within four days, the Sheriffs Department showed up with a court order to have me committed back into the hospital. Apparently, this was brought about by a court action initiated by Sandy. I had been in my townhouse bothering or seeing no one but a couple of close friends. Needless to say, I was extremely angry, hurt and embarrassed by my sister's actions.

The two deputies that transported me to the hospital knew me well, along with my outstanding reputation in the community. They assured me that I would only be detained at the hospital a few minutes. They refused to return to LaGrange until after I had met with the Medical Director. I immediately saw the doctor, and he informed me that he didn't like this court action taken by my sister, but he indicated to me that he was required to hold me a minimum of five days. He did, however, assure me that I would not be held a minute longer than the law required.

Sandy told mother that she was sure those were my drugs in my truck, and that she was sure that I would soon be arrested if I didn't get help. The doctor assured me that he knew it was not my bag of cocaine and had to have been planted. The doctor immediately informed me that Sandy could be imprisoned for three years and fined $10,000 for committing me when I was absolutely no danger to anyone or myself. The court order stated that I was suicidal and a danger to those around me, but the doctor said there was absolutely no truth to those claims. Needless to say, it was a long and angry five days.

However, the doctor did indeed release me on the hour.

Upon returning home, I soon learned that Sandy had requested ten percent of the corporate stock. Needing her at this point, I agreed to this, knowing she had lied all along.

The man suspected of planting drugs in my truck was soon arrested. One of the many charges pending against this man was planting illegal drugs in someone else's vehicle. I began to read my Bible each night until I had completely read the entire fascinating book.

By this time, my sister seemed to have taken sole charge of my business affairs, making me feel as if I wasn't really needed. After this experience and two hospital visits, I felt very inferior and depressed. I was to be like this for the next eighteen long months.

On one of my few visits to my restaurants, I was in noticeable extreme pain from my previously broken neck. A fine Christian lady who had worked for me the past two years approached me saying, "You need help and I have this fine Christian doctor that can indeed help you." She said that the doctors at the Hughston Clinic were JFK's old doctors as well as special doctors for the National Football League. I learned that this hospital was located in nearby Columbus, Georgia, and that they had performed back surgery on her. I called the clinic immediately and got my first appointment within two short weeks.

After two weeks on an unsuccessful medication, the doctor stated that the only alternative was surgery to fuse my spine. He wanted to put me in the hospital on January 27, 1982, which was my birthday. We agreed on January 28.

Prior to my surgery, my mother came up not only to be with me but along with Sandy's insistence to persuade me to move to Tallahassee immediately following surgery. I knew Sandy wanted me completely away from my business, but I also felt a great need to be near my children in Tallahassee. Reluctantly, I gave in once more. Sandy assured me that she would run the business "as if it were her own," and always continue to send me my same monthly check. She also agreed to manage my moving to Tallahassee after surgery. I was soon to find out that 1982 would be another horrible year, as was 1980.

Sandy had kept, and would keep, her power of attorney over me.

They operated on January 29, and I came out of surgery in extreme pain. I remained in the hospital for another six days and returned to LaGrange with my mother to close out my bank accounts. I then moved in with my mother in Tallahassee until I was well enough to get an apartment. The pain was excruciating for another three weeks as I was having terrible migraine headaches due to the surgery performed on my spine.

After the migraines were gone, I took the first apartment I looked at. I was still extremely weak at this time. However, I had regained much of my strength during the week it took my furniture to arrive. There was little I could do now but recover, which would take months of daily rest and continuous twenty-four-hour wearing of my most uncomfortable neck brace. However, recovery became much easier as I began once again to see my children on a regular basis.

I rested each day and began to go out several nights a week meeting many good-looking women. I found myself going out seven nights a week just to entertain most of them. Somehow none of these ten women knew about each other. I've never had such luck! I guess, with my brace, they felt sorry for me at first and then became attracted to me. However, after a couple of months, I became burned out and most unhappy with my playboy image and settled down to the two women I seemed to have strong feelings for. They soon found out about each other, but only due to my honesty.

In May of the same year, I had my children one weekend and also had an important engagement with my date. I never enjoyed leaving my children with a sitter but I felt compelled to attend this engagement, so I hired one. I soon came to believe that the sitter had brought severe bodily and mental harm to my then three-and-one-half-year old son. I became very angry and once again in a manic state. I was immediately able to contact an authority on the subject, and it was this professional's opinion that my son receive much loving care, some therapy, and that the sitter be turned over to the authorities.

I made the mistake of approaching my mother with my findings. She told me I was manic and needed help again. She asked me to do nothing for twenty-four hours and I returned the next day as she had requested. She then informed me that I could voluntarily check myself into the hospital for a few days or she would commit me because I was insane to think of my own sitter in this way.

I voluntarily entered the hospital being assured that I could stay the three days I felt I needed to calm down. Unfortunately, I was put on the closed ward where I was put on heavy doses of drugs which soon turned me into a complete zombie. The doctors never addressed the question nor mentioned the incident with my nephew and son which put me into this manic condition. I was in the hospital for three days and they refused to allow me to leave, saying that I was in need of additional treatment. Of course, during the first three days, I received no therapy only heavy doses of drugs.

Several days later, I had a patient attack me, shoving a fork to my throat and saying he was going to cut out my jugular vein. To avoid a fight, I ran into the staff office where five male staff members were laughing and joking. When I cried out for help they immediately jumped on me and began beating me up. I told them I had recently had spinal surgery on my neck, and please don't hurt me. This big black BoZo took my neck and almost twisted it off, as if he were attempting to re-break it. I was told to get off the floor but as I stood, I was in excruciating pain in both my neck and shoulder. In fact, I couldn't raise my right arm or shoulder at all. I soon wished I had taken my chances with the loony with the fork. When I asked the staff members why I was beat up, they just laughed and escorted me to the box or isolation hole. I remained there for three days without ever seeing a doctor. When released from the hole, there was still no explanation given for their treatment to me. I was unable to raise my right arm or shoulder for three months even to brush my teeth. They simply told my mother that I had a freak accident and fell to the floor.

Ten clays after this horrible incident, I was still a zombie against my will, due to the heavy doses of drugs given to me. Soon some friends I had attended church with for twenty years came into the visiting room. I assumed that they were there to visit me, so I approached them calling them by name and shaking hands. I was immediately dragged away from my friends, who happened to be there to visit someone else and unaware that I was also there. As they dragged me away, it became apparent they didn't want anyone to know just how drugged I was or how they were treating me. They immediately threw me back in the hole and made me beg and beg to go to the restroom. I felt as though I was in a prison camp. I was, however, released from the hole later that day with absolutely no explanation as to why I was even locked up for merely speaking to some church friends.

Within the next couple of days, I began to feel as though my medication had been increased. I became a total zombie and distinctly recall asking why my mother hadn't visited me in several days, only to be told by a staff member that "she was dead."

At 7:00 a.m. the next morning, I was very angry and acquired the use of a phone, only to call the administrator of the parent hospital at his home. I explained my situation and treatment here and requested a badly needed meeting with this man. He assured me that he would notify his secretary to do so if I would phone his office after 9:00 a.m. Other than the two of us, no one knew of this phone call. Within an hour, he must have phoned this facility because I was locked up in the hole again, reportedly "for making an inappropriate phone call." I remained in the hole for one day.

The next two days I planned my escape from this tight-security facility. At the right time on the second day, I put my devious escape plan into action. I made it 100 yards from the facility before being recaptured.

Two staff members who knew me from high school approached me saying they agreed with my complaint of abuse and neglect. These friends informed me that I was now to be given heavy doses of Haidol and lithium together. I knew from previous experience that taking these two drugs together can be fatal. I was told by these two insiders simply not to swallow the medication. They said that the doctors feared I would blow the lid off the facility; and if patients weren't ready for release within two weeks, they were transferred to the state hospital as this was only a short-term treatment facility. They told me that I had already been kept here eight weeks because they were afraid I would talk if I transferred anywhere else. They said this in strict confidence and asked me to repeat it to no one for fear they might lose their jobs. Needless to say, I began to swallow only the lithium and spit out the Haldol and everything else. Very soon, I began to feel and look much better.

One morning I had a brief and startling conference with some doctor who said he had the ideal treatment for me in a hospital in Georgia. He said that I would receive some funny drugs and treatments which would make me forget all I had been through. I knew this had to be shock treatment since I knew they were illegal in the State of Florida. I immediately said, "Sure, then I can easily collect two-million dollars from you and this hospital for prescribing a dangerous and unnecessary shock treatment." Extremely angry, I got up and immediately left his office. When I turned to say good-bye, I observed a baffled look of dismay.

My mother was beginning to realize that my treatment was less than good here. On one of her visits, she said that she had some very good news. She told me that through the help of our local U.S. senator and friends, she had arranged for me to be transferred to a facility in Maryland as soon as there was an opening. I knew this must be a good hospital, as she said this was where all the congressmen and senators are hospitalized.

With the help of the United States government, they realized that I possibly wouldn't be able to be kept quiet, or even from filing suit. Therefore, I was soon transferred to the open ward where I had more room and privacy along with the use of a pay telephone. My medication had been cut back. There were still an awful lot of extremely dangerous patients on open ward, and I remained angry at my prior levels of medication and abusive treatment.

Within the next two days, I began to make some powerful and damaging phone calls against this hospital. I phoned my spinal doctor in Georgia to discuss my abusive treatment along with my recent neck and shoulder injury. I then wasted no time in calling the investigative unit of the state of Florida.

As a result of these two calls, frequent investigations were made by the state agency. Needless to say, the doctors were very upset and disturbed at my actions. In fact, the doctor even went so far as to say that I would not be allowed to go to N.I.H. I immediately said, "You and this little hospital of yours can't refuse to turn me over to the United States government," and walked out of his office very angry, knowing I had yet more to do.

I figure that if this doctor was going to attempt to defy the U.S. Government, I would make one more damaging phone call. I phoned the Jacksonville Federal Bureau of Investigation Headquarters later that evening explaining just what they had done to me and the extensive use of drugs on many of the patients. I spoke to an agent here at some length and he assured me that they would investigate these charges immediately.

Arrivals had always come in slowly, maybe in the mornings or maybe in the evenings. However, this next morning four new patients arrived. Three appeared to be quite well and one appeared to be very messed up, and hung over. He wore only one sock and no shoes.

I noticed that the three well patients seemed to spend much time together conversing, and occasionally talking to the hung over patient. I immediately got to know these individuals, attempting to find out if they could have been sent in to investigate by the Federals. They seemed rather reserved with their information but did reveal that they were all former military. One, in fact, worked at the Pentagon in Washington, D.C. As well as they appeared and spoke, I was convinced that they were here to investigate on behalf of the FBI, I left this inner circle to follow this hung over one awhile. It was 2:00 p.m., and he was still appearing to be hung over, and he was still walking around with only one sock on. He approached each severely drugged patient saying, "Hi! Gee, I'm coming down, and I need some of what you got! Next time you get your medication, tell me the color and number on your pill." He did this to each patient who appeared to be heavily drugged and then approached the inner circle of the other three. I knew then by his stable appearance and distant but apparent "Faking it," he must have had considerable pharmaceutical training. These other three for two mornings literally ran and controlled our morning "joke meeting" between staff and patients. They would make statements such as "Why complain? There is no doctor or medical doctor here to answer our complaints," Both meetings lasted no more than five minutes.

Within thirty-six hours this hospital made a complete turnaround in patient care, and had eliminated totally its policy of excessive drug use on patients. In fact, most patients were now being given nothing more than a daily vitamin pill. To my astonishment all forty of these new arrivals had departed, as had quite a few other patients who had no business in this facility. It was extremely rare. I have never seen such a quick departure by anyone from such a facility.

I was allowed to change to a doctor of my choice, Dr. A. After reviewing my records and after several conversations with me and family, he simply said he felt my family made me manic. He, along with two previous doctors in Georgia, believed that I didn't even need lithium. However, he did say that he would continue the lithium, but I would be much better off if I could avoid my family. Dr. A. assured me that I would be leaving on a flight to NIH within a week. I was nowhere near manic and only wished that I could just be discharged, but I guess the hospital was afraid who I would talk to further. I had pretty well ruined the name of this facility already, what with the press talk of building a new and better facility.

Within five days, my wonderful and loving sister, Cindy, and her husband, Jim, arrived at 5:00 a.m. to pick me up for our flight to NIH in Maryland. I was so glad to get away from this terrible facility but I knew I would never forget the horrible treatment and abuse I had received. After all these investigations I had initiated, the patient load was only half of its capacity.

I was well greeted and received with prompt attention at NIH. The facility was nice and comfortable and not crowded at all. The patient limit was eight and all manics. However, the following day to my dismay, I discovered the staff and my doctor wanted me to stay for six months for some new experimental testing on manics. I thought about it for a couple of days and discussed these treatments with the patients who were currently undergoing them. One patient informed me that they stuck needles in your eyes for one of those new tests. Having been blinded once in my life, I then decided that I was going to leave this place somehow.

Still in much pain from being maliciously mauled by those five staff members of Goodwood Manor, I requested x-rays for my neck and shoulder. Upon x-raying my neck and shoulders, a specialist informed me that there had indeed been some damage to my neck, and he recommended that I return to the spinal clinic in Georgia, as soon as possible.

In meeting with the doctor and staff the next day, they informed me that they would release me but they would have to release me back to "Badtree Manor." I reluctantly said yes, and was assured that they would arrange me an escort, and flight back to Tallahassee. I had stayed a total of ten days before my flight departed. I was assured by my NIH escort that Goodwood Manor would receive a good report on me and further recommend an early release.

Upon returning to the Goodwood Manor something was extremely strange-I didn't see any patients. Later, I learned that there were only four patients left with a patient capacity of forty-eight. Prior to my excessive phone use and subsequent investigations, the hospital was always filled at or near capacity. I immediately found out that I would be seeing a friend of Dr. C, and not Dr. A. Dr. S was assigned to my case because he prepared the paperwork on my NIH trip and was there to receive my report from NIH escort. After much persuasion, I was kept here in this empty hospital for five days before I was finally released. My mom was happy that I was out, but not happy that I had left NIH. I told her that I just could not face being locked up another six months for the benefit of a scientific study.

By now, I had not only lost my great wealth, I had lost my dignity for having been locked up and treated like an animal for five months.

My problems in the past with my mother were due to the fact that my doctor was in contact with her and my ex-wife whenever I came near a manic condition. This is, of course, against all medical ethics and would only fuel me into a full blown manic condition rather than permit the doctor's private and confidential ability to bring me out of this high.

In less than fourteen months, I was in a high once again, and began investing heavily in what I had considered a sound investment with some business associates of mine. When I told Mother of these investments, she immediately became angry. Needless to say, I went into a milder but still manic condition once again. She spoke to Dr. W., at great length insisting that "something be done," though I felt I was completely harmless to anyone. At first, she insisted and later demanded that I check into Behavioral Medical Care (BMC). She further insisted that if I didn't, she would get a court order. I asked, "On what grounds?" She said, "Jim, you are in a manic condition!" I replied, "Sure, I'm around you, but once I leave I'll come down, because your lack of understanding makes me manic."

I had a bank job at this time and had received nothing but praise from my superiors. Furthermore, I told her that someone is not locked up just for being manic unless they are a danger to society or self She still demanded, and reluctantly I gave in knowing she would indeed get a court order.

Upon arriving at BMC, I realized it was no more than the horrible Goodwood Manor with a new name and the same doctors. I am sure they changed their name due to the bad publicity they had received on my behalf

I was put on the open ward but was most unhappy with the treatment I was receiving from Dr. S. After he told me I would be there for sometime, I said, "Simply because I can't get along with my mother? Because I certainly function well with everyone else." I then demanded a court hearing and got it in a matter of days. The hearing was a joke. Dr. S. referred to me as unstable and paranoid. They immediately left to avoid any cross examination by my dear friend and attorney, Joe Jacobs, who had known me well for twenty years and insisted these accusations were not true. As for myself, I informed the Judge that I was very stable and was definitely not paranoid, nor did Dr. S. state what I was paranoid about. The Judge believed the untruths of the departed doctor who refused to answer any of the questions. He sentenced me to six months in Florida State Hospital. I was angry and upset to have experienced such a "monkey trial," but I was happy to get away from this same old treatment and Dr. S.

At the state hospital I received excellent treatment along with my side of the story being heard. My doctor, and entire team of counselors, and social workers, believed I did not belong in this or any hospital simply because I couldn't get along with my mother. They assured me that I would only be in the hospital two to three weeks to give them time to re-evaluate me and have the Judge's Court Order overruled. My counselor later informed me that I should contact the state attorney's office along with the attorney general and bring charges against the Tallahassee hospital and its doctors for my treatment in 1982 as well as my recent treatment,

On their word, I was soon released to my mother's total shock and amazement. The doctors and team reminded me that I never belonged here nor did they ever want to see me or hear of me being locked up again.

At the time of my release, it was about one week before Christmas of 1983 which I had no desire to spend with my mother. I rushed and bought my kids their Christmas presents and visited them, and then took off for Newberry, South Carolina, to visit my dear grandmother. She spoke very much of Dad as I listened patiently learning much I had never known about him and what a hero he was during World War II. We spent a quiet yet wonderful Christmas together filled with a lot of snow to bring about the Christmas spirit. After Christmas, I returned to Tallahassee to rebuild my life once again.

I returned to Dr. W. as he was practicing at the free county clinic and my funds were somewhat low. I saw Dr. W. once every three months for three-and-one-half years with no problem and without even coming close to a manic condition. I did, however, have another serious problem in my life. Since the Goodwood Manor incident my neck had become extremely painful.

By 1985, I was once again under the knife undergoing two more spinal fusions at the Hugston Clinic. It would once again take me months to recover along with constant wearing of my neck brace. I felt only a 20% reduction in pain this time and would find out my disc would degenerate even more. In February of '87, I was back on the operating table for the most critical surgery I had feared. I was to be wired and fused in five additional places in my neck. Prior to the surgery, I was a nervous wreck, very fearful of being paralyzed after. I required the constant companionship of a dear lady friend to see me through this difficult time. As with the two previous spinal operations, the first thing I did after awakening was to move my legs with joy and praise the Lord. Following this rather extensive surgery, I was in much more pain and in an uncomfortable neck brace twenty-four hours a day. I soon developed a bad infection and blood clot in my neck along with a 104 degree temperature. At this writing, my neck is, however, experiencing a good 30-35% less pain.

In June, I returned to the Bahamas after ten years and had a great time. I drank entirely too much but never got drunk. I hadn't been drinking very often at all, but the atmosphere of being on a cruise with everyone else drinking and the constant party atmosphere enticed me to drink too much. At that time I was manic and should have realized it would lower my lithium level. I had so much fun on both the ship and the islands that I became hyperverbal and upon returning home occasionally felt hypermanic but definitely not manic.

At this time, I began to think about it being an appropriate time to file for joint custody of my children. I met with my attorney who said I had a good to excellent chance. I requested Health and Rehabilitative Services to investigate both my ex-wife and me and give an opinion to the court concerning what would be best for the children's welfare. (I also included my mother in the investigation.)

My three months had elapsed since I had seen Dr. W., and I entered the clinic to meet with my counselor. Right off, I told her I was hyperverbal and that my mother was once again alarmed. The counselor agreed that I was indeed hyperverbal but stated that she would be too if she had just gotten back from the Bahamas. She also assured me that I was not hypermanic or manic, nor had she ever seen me in these conditions in the four years she had been counseling me. After seeing Sadie, I went into Dr. W's office for a brief visit. At that time, he said that I was becoming manic. Thus, I had to start seeing Dr. W., and my counselor, Ms. S., three times a week. In two days. I returned and Ms. S. told me that my ex-wife had spoken to Dr. W., and both she and my mother were extremely upset with my Health and Rehabilitative Services inquiry into their lives.

After seeing Ms. S., I again saw Dr. W., who told me that I was manic and to stay out of my ex-wife's life. He then reached into his desk drawer and came up with eleven pills for me to swallow. (Note: Ms. S. had just seen me and said I wasn't manic.) The next morning I was again horrified to open my door and find two deputies with a court order for my hospitalization. The court order read that I was suicidal and not taking my medication. Although it was an absurd lie, I had no choice but to go with them. Once again, I received a message from above saying: "Son, I, the Almighty and your Lord and Savior, will protect and defend you; go with these men for you will not be locked up." I felt but did not reveal this confidence I had received from above as I entered yet another institution.

I was sure that this court order had been initiated by my ex-wife who was now an attorney and her friend Dr. W. I also knew that I had to hold back my anger toward these two. One deputy remained at the facility claiming I appeared fine, that he was sure they would not keep me and he would remain to give me a ride home.

I first met with a counselor by the name of Mike, who was rude and argumentative when I asked him his title and qualifications. I later met with a Dr. 0., who was reportedly the head psychiatrist. I found him to be very friendly and informed on the subject of manic depression. He indicated that he felt I was not suicidal and seemed concerned about my medication level. He seemed satisfied that I had taken my medication and stated that he was not going to commit or allow me to stay in this facility because he felt placement was inappropriate. I thanked God for his protection against such injustice as I returned home again.

That evening I attempted to speak to my children by phone but was refused.

The next day I met Ms. S., my counselor at the clinic for what I thought would be a normal twenty-minute session, Ms. S. told me she was sorry for what I had been through the day before, but that she had arranged for me to interview the doctor and three manic patients, who would provide valuable information for this book. I immediately became suspicious but was assured by her that I could leave any time I wanted and that there would be no tricks. Ms. S. gave me a pen and pad to take notes on for the book. Since Ms. S. assured me I would not be locked up, I proceeded next door to the hospital psychiatric unit to find a rude and arrogant Dr. H. instead of the friendly Dr. 0. He informed me to get all the notes I wanted from the patients as he was finished with me, and further, I could not leave the hospital until I was ready.

As I was marched off, I looked at Ms. S., saying: "You lied! You tricked me!" I was once again locked up in an institution.

I knew that the previous court order had been dismissed by Dr. 0., and there wasn't a new court order, so my rights were being totally violated. Furthermore, I had just been to my attorney's office, who knew my and other manics' condition quite well, and he mentioned nothing about my being manic.

The first day, all I could think about was why God would save me from injustice as he said he would, only to forsake me the next day. I knew by that evening that God didn't work that way, as some things just happen and God gives us freedom not by controlling our life-events but by showing us how to handle and deal with these events and tragedies.

The next morning I saw Dr. 0 and I felt as if his hands had been tied because he had very little to say to me as opposed to the previous day when he was most helpful. I felt as though young Dr. 0. did not have sufficient influence over the older and arrogant Dr. H. to release me without obtaining additional help. Therefore, I requested a hearing to determine that my rights had indeed been violated and that I should be released. I was held there more than the legal five days without a hearing, once again violating my rights. I phoned the public defender's office and was assured by them that I would have a hearing in three days, only to watch three days go by. The next morning I saw Dr. 0., and he indicated to me that they had decided to release me very soon.

I figured, however, since Dr. H. had no valid right to have locked the doors behind me on my visit, no judge in Tallahassee was willing to hear such a fraudulent case. Within a week my sister Cindy arrived to pick me up, as Dr. 0 was releasing me on the thirteenth day of my illegal incarceration. I explained to Dr. 0. that I was most unhappy with Dr. W. and his breach of patient confidentiality with both my mother and ex-wife. Dr. 0. advised against a state doctor and suggested I find a good doctor that I could afford to pay for. When I got in the car with my sister, she informed me that Dr. 0. had told her he had to release me, or the hospital would be faced with a large lawsuit

I had been able to refrain from an angry manic attitude toward Dr. 0, as I was not angry at him at all. However, after twenty-one horrible days of illegal incarceration, I had become somewhat manic due to my anger toward Dr. H., along with Dr. W., who even on the last day was there insisting Dr. 0. not release me. I'm sure that my ex-wife was continuing to burn up the phone with her influence.

Therefore, I went home, packed my suitcase and left town for the coast by late afternoon to avoid any possible future action by my wife and Dr. W. Near sundown, there was no motel around; I remembered, however, my old friend Doug, who had a large beach cottage nearby. I told Doug my bizarre story. Doug informed me that I was manic and found my story hard to believe. I agreed that I was manic as I had very little sleep for those twenty-one days due to the constant yelling and talking of patients each night. I asked him to allow me to stay over for a night and sleep, and allow myself to come down the next day. Well, manics, don't always expect your friends to help you when you desperately need them. Doug deeply hurt me by saying no.

Feeling very rejected and devastated by this lack of compassion and understanding, I walked to my car feeling as though I didn't have a friend in the world but the Lord himself.

My lithium level was a perfect 1.0. 1, only needed a friend to help me overcome this ordeal I had been through. Furthermore, if he had seen me through this ordeal, the even worse danger and horror I was soon to face would have been avoided. To make matters even worse, I found out later that Doug had phoned my mother, which alarmed her.

Feeling very rejected, I drove down the coast until I found a small motel out in the boondocks. I was most unhappy with the miserable conditions but stayed there for a week attempting to overcome my anger without a friend in the world to talk to in this desolate place.

After a week, I left this retreat hoping to find a more suitable and relaxing environment to allow me to come down before returning home. This never happened. A sheriff pulled up beside me as I parked at a bank and requested that I get into the back seat of the squad car for a ride to the county jail. There, I was questioned by a psychiatrist, and I knew I had been set up by someone who felt that I needed to be removed from the streets again. There was no mention of any violation or why I was picked up. I was hyper during this questioning but never manic, nor did I in any way feel dangerous to anyone or to myself.

I never did see a court order stating the reasons but I was taken to a hospital in Panama City and placed on the mental ward. I told no one where my mother lived or her phone number, yet she knew where I was, which only proves someone I knew had arranged to have me picked up. I was very angry and even sometimes manic due to my needless incarceration. I requested and even demanded a hearing within the legal five-day trial limit.

I received a ten minute psychological evaluation by a Dr. H. In thirteen days I was allowed to go before a judge who seemed to be very attentive to the lying doctor. I had earlier told this doctor that I had been wired and put back together in a dozen places along with the fact that I somewhat previously had been under FBI protective custody. She took these statements and twisted them to say I had told her "I was wired to a computer and was now working for the CIA" along with several other false statements to this judge. I had earlier criticized Dr. C's treatment of me in 1982 to the judge and later to the patients when I heard his name mentioned, only to find out that he also worked in this mental ward. I figured that the judge must want to cover for the doctor by setting me up for six months in the state hospital.

Needless to say, I was devastated at being transferred the next morning and was placed in a ward with some very strange, sick, violent and insane patients. I was on a closed ward and had a new doctor (Dr. E). This was a lady doctor who completed her fifteen minute pre-admission psychological evaluation upon my arrival. I then saw her three minutes a week thereafter. She increased my lithium to between 1900-2 100 milligrams without considering the fact that I was never able to tolerate the side effects of over 900 milligrams. She also started me on heavy doses of mellaril--800 mg. a day. Thus, immediately I began to feel drunk and sleepy. (I did not swallow the daytime doses.)

As has always been the case, I was very well liked by most of the patients and this was disturbing to the rough and violent ones who made it quite clear we would soon be fighting each other. I explained what was about to happen to both my team and doctor and requested to be moved to the much quieter and less populated open ward for my safety. After my weekly three minutes with Dr. E, were up, I was told that they would think about it. I had been an extremely well-behaved patient for three weeks and was very disappointed when my transfer request was turned down. I knew that fighting for my own life was certain.

Within the next week, I settled four bad situations without fight-ing only to be involved in four fights I could not avoid. In one of these fights, I fought for the second time an angry animal who had once killed another man. In this fight I nearly lost my left eye as he attempted to snatch it out, later to only laugh when I was going to the emergency room for treatment and on to an eye specialist. I did not lose any of my fights but did not receive any satisfaction out of fighting. In each report, it was documented to my team and doctor that I did not start, nor could I have avoided, either fight. I thought for sure, after my serious eye injury, I would be transferred to an open ward. This would not happen for another two days when several team members and my doctor observed a wild patient who started swinging angrily at me for no reason. I avoided all punches and grabbed him as did the staff and was then approached by my doctor and documented for trying to avoid the fight. Within several hours, I was transferred to the quieter and less populated open war.

I was given outside privileges which I cherished and began to once again feel God's presence as I was outside. I knew that God was within my heart and soul, but I couldn't feel his presence in the devil-infected building except in my own heart--definitely not in my surroundings.

My next privilege was that of a weekend pass to spend with my mother. I went to football games with friends and dates, as well as other social activities and had no problem except the horror of returning to the locked doors at the hospital. My doctor after about four weekend passes informed me that I would be released after one or two more successful visits home. To my total shock and disappointment, I was transferred to a new unit and building only to have a new team and doctor who needed to get to know me. I soon learned that I had a fine Christian doctor as well as a Christian team who admired my strong religious beliefs. I had felt no Christianity within the hearts of my previous doctor and team. After reviewing my records and evaluating me, my new doctor (Dr. A) said: "I don't understand why you are here, and we will do our best to have you released in the next few weeks." I was given a weekend pass and then an eleven-day leave pass. I returned only to be released permanently the following morning. I spent a night here.

Over three months of my life was once again taken from me, and I was never told by anyone that I was a danger to society or myself, which should be the only reason an individual can be incarcerated in a mental institution.

In 1990, I decided to take a vacation by myself because I was never allowed to take my children on vacation. Upon returning to

Tallahassee, I picked up a hitchhiker named Mike. I later found out that he was an alcoholic and a criminal. When we stopped at an intersection for a red light, he jumped out of the car and went around to the driver's side and opened the car door and threw me out of the vehicle and stole my car. I ran to a nearby convenience store to use the phone, and he proceeded up the street in my car. I called 911 from the phone inside the store. Unknown to me, my mother had taken out a warrant for me under the Baker act. While I was still on the phone to police dispatch, the officers came up to me, threw down my suitcase and searched it, and, then, for no good reason, beat me with night sticks. I was taken to the emergency room at Tallahassee Memorial Regional Medical Center, patched up, and then taken to the new TMRMC Psychiatric Center. As usual, I was put in a closed ward. My roommate was a murderer. I knew I was trapped. I asked for my suitcase, medications and my Bible. The police did let me have my Bible, Thank God.

The next morning, I was up early and called my mother. She told me she didn't think the car was stolen because bottles were found in the vehicle, and she thought I had been drinking. I had not. The bottles had belonged to Mike, the hitchhiker.

I prayed that I could contact President Bush. I opened the Bible and found his telephone number. Since I was an original founder of The Republican Congressional Select Committee, my call was immediately accepted. The personal secretary told me that she already knew exactly where I was, and they were concerned about me. At that point, the hospital medical staff took the phone from me. I told them I could call anyone I wanted to call because I knew how the government worked and was well aware of the First Amendment to tile Constitution. I was told never to call him again. The staff then wrestled me to the floor. I was so shocked and amazed that this could happen. I started crying. Only one nurse showed any concern. She later came to me and took me outside for a cigarette. She told me she was a retired navy nurse and that she was undercover and would look out for me.

I don't remember all the doctors who attended me before I was released, but I remembered one in particular - Dr. Chocawala, who finally gave me open yard privileges, and one day I was lying on a table to get my back comfortable. A beautiful yellow tiger swallow tail butterfly landed right in the palm of my hand, and as I looked up, there was Dr. Chocawala. Within one hour, I was taken to a closed ward - taken back only because God's creature came to me and was lighting up the world outside for the other patients, as I was drawing a crowd.

To sum up a long story, I finally got out in about a month. Dr. S. who, like Dr. Chocawala was a Buddhist from India, released me on a dangerous drug called Tegratol, which made me sleepy all the time. I went back to my miserable little apartment. Then, I returned to Dr. Eckwall for treatment.

It's good to know that President Bush loved me so much. President Bush requested a pass be given to me for me to visit him in the White House. He also called Dr. Rev. Billy Graham to pray for me on nationwide live radio address. However, they would not totally release me to the President of the United States Government.

In January 199 1, my mother died. She jut blew up with a brain tumor. She had two brain tumors. I continuously took her to the hospital for treatments and tried to keep her alive. She died within six months of reading my book.

The only time I had been sent back to the horrible Florida State Hospital since my mother died was in January 1992, and the power chain went to work, and a lady doctor got me out within two weeks. I then went to a halfway house. Previously, Dr. Esguta tied me down by all fours for two weeks, just because a patient tried to kill me. I did not even throw a punch. It was extremely painful on my neck and spine.

I proceeded to call CBS News in New York and talked with Dan Rather. He suggested I go on "60 Minutes," as I had too big of a story that should be told. Mr. Rather then picked up the phone and ordered a copy of my book, and I got a letter stating that he had received his copy.

I have, however, been locked up several times by organized crime in Tallahassee, where you have no rights, or telephone. It's a pri-vately-owned hospital. Dr. Hebron remembered me, and said she couldn't be my doctor because of organized crime. Otherwise, she would let me go. I have been held here sometimes for over 60 days for such things as trying to help a half-blind lady get some food. One of her jealous relatives called the law on me.

I do have an awful lot of undercover friends who work at Eastside Hospital. The problem with most doctors in Tallahassee is that they are imported foreign doctors. They are Buddhist or atheist, and do not believe in God. Also, the Florida Constitution conflicts with the U.S. Constitution period.

I'm highly allergic and react adversely to dangerous drugs issued by Eastside and their foreign doctors. The Eastside facility, where I've been locked up several times, had two special doctors

Dr. Mejia. He is no longer there. He's now a private psychiatrist and M.D., and, in fact, I was his first patient. However, he is now leaving the State of Florida, and I have no idea who I can trust. He would tell me, while at Eastside Hospital, that nothing was wrong with my head and he would release me in several days after observ-ing me Dr. Mejia, who is Spanish, tells me I was a fine patient and a better psychiatrist, sometimes, than he is. He knows the PDR book well. Dr. Mejia's title is not psychiatrist - he is Dr. Mejia, M.D., Gen-eral Psychiatry. He knows I am in pain, and does not want me locked up. He is a good friend. He has even invited me to his home. Many psychiatrists think they're better than you. The Bible says nobody is better than anyone else. Wisdom, knowledge and the truth shall over-come.

The other good doctor I had at Eastside was Dr. Alenzuela this two years prior to releasing this book. After being there several days, he stated I was not sick or mentally ill, but just irritated, which I should be.

The most terrible thing in my life is when I lost my father in 1980. Losing his job as Budget Director of Florida HRS was a great loss to the State. And, furthermore, he would have never let me suffer a day, much less 15 years.

Secretary of HRS, O.J. Keller, was fired by Governor Martinez. Keller was director of HRS, and also a friend of mine, and my dad's boss. HRS had fallen apart, and nobody investigates the institutions like they should, and it's required by the Federal government. And, like my Daddy and I did most of our lives, we worked with many governors.

I was chosen to head up a committee for RRS by the government. And, the title of the book was "Delivering Human Services," and I made most of the suggestions for this book, and it was destroyed when my Daddy died. All my troubles with my enemies started,.

One of the most disappointing times in my life was when my children refused to accept me as I was. This lasted for approximately two years or more. In fact, it was devastating to me. However, much has changed, they no long ignore or avoid me. They correspond with me up here in Georgia and they and their mother do good deeds for me-God bless them.

Thank you and may God bless you and enrich our lives, so we can help those less fortunate than we are. Amen!

CHAPTER XI

Evaluating Medically...

Of James O. Wessinger III

by

Nurse/Author

Ms. Coucinda McKeon

This is part of my medical report prepared for the judge by a very qualified nurse, Lucinda McKeon—also an author herself— who constantly observed me in and out of the hospital. It was never presented to the judge, as my attorney felt it would destroy my soon-to-be ex-wife, Barbara.

My main purpose in conglomerating facts medically here, is surely urgent and severely important for superiors to read and comprehend thoroughly. I believe that possibly, Jim will have to try, once again, to defend his mental capabilities...and this is where I am trying to make visual for you to realize the obvious and conjunctured past that Jim has been coping with for sometime. There is no demoralizing on my part or Jim's, for anyone involved. We are simply correlating-- together, his past experience and my knowledge and studies on psychology, human behavior, and most importantly, my parmochology education from the state of Georgia. I, of course, am no expert, and far from qualified personally to ever judge and/or be diagnosing another human being...there, I am offering you my medical books them printed and adopted statements...and somewhere along each important statement (to me), I have my opinion. It may be irrelevant, nevertheless, I am not incorrect, and all I'm asking is, please ready and consider all the possibilities of a slow process of dementalizing the mind of a successful, proprius, or complex (yet simple too) business man...that has bordered him to destruction — a couple of times — but never succeeded in beating the truth.

I now sincerely hope this information will not be illegible to you and too, that it will become the key, ambeitn tool for justice.

All Medical References Used:

Clinical Pharmacology- (Lippincott-Scherer)-pp. 241-243
Psychiatric Nursing 3rd Edition- (Sturt-Sundeen)-pp. 260-314
Understanding Human Behavior (Milliken-Delmar)-pp. 100-113
Psychiatric Nursing- 2nd Edition- (Burgess-Lazare)--pp. 203-283
Encyclopedia and Dictionary of Medicine-2nd Edition (Miller-Keane)-pp. 840-841
Pharmacology in Nuring Interventions (Bergersen) pp. 294
PDR-Physicians Desk Reference

PSYCHOSIS:

Jim has always faced his problems and talked about them...and opened his mind continuingly for advice.

Because of the Major Drug that Jim was placed on last year and\ ministered to him by his wife-Barbara. I do NOT believe she was qualified to give such an important sedative, with many known contraindication and many unknown side-effects. And too, this drug is prescribed to psychotic patients that should be monitored hourly for precautions, and altered with the dosages periodically

I know this was not performed ... and Jim did have a reverse reaction and almost died. Strangely enough, he has managed to survive this whole circular, unorganized, and fraudulent life style, he has lived in for quite sometime now.

At any rate, this is why I am opening all medical doors for physical and mental evaluational concepts, for yall to please consider, and discuss. If it is a question ever arising in this debation of Jim's mental status I will stand and fight for him- because I know he is capable of handling...Today.

Medications commonly used in manic depressives

(contraindicions-side effects-adverse reactions) -may be listed and please NOTE if available to reach an un-medical and conclusive decision in just what is being questioned here!

Medications commonly used in psychiatry

Psychopharmacotherapy therapy is a specialized field that is presently involved in a knowledge explosion. Research is being conducted in many areas and information about medications seems to expand and change every day. Nurses need to be aware of important developments in this field One way to accomplish this is by regularly literature particularly periodicals. Pharmacists are good resource people and can recommend helpful research reports or can assist in evaluation of conflicting research findings. Information provided by pharmaceutical companies should be used with discrimination; it may be valid, but they rarely disseminate findings that reflect negatively on their product.

This section is not an attempt to provide exhaustive information on psychotropic medications. Interested readers may find such information in great detail in pharmacology texts. The focus here will be to delineate the major categories Of medication commonly prescribed for psychiatric patients and the most frequently encountered nursing implications. These are all powerful drugs and may cause responses that have not been mentioned here.

Trade name	Dosage	Dose form
Haidol	2 to 15	Tablet
Tegrarol	200-1000 mg,	Tablet
Lithium	300-15000 mg,	Capsule

Side Effects:
Overseduation impaired psychomotor functions, akathisia. Parkinson syndrome, dystonia, orthostatic hypotension, anticholinergic effects, impotence, photosensitivity, weight gain, lactation, menstrual irregularity, potentiation of other drugs and alcohol

Complications:
Tardive dyskinesia seizures, cholestatic jaundice, agranulocytosis rash, pigmentary eye change (chiorpromazine and thioridazine only).

Any concern expressed by a patient about medication should be taken seriously and reported to the physician. The major categories of medications that will be discussed are (1) the antipsychotic agents (2) the antianxiety agents, (3) the antidepressants, and (4) lithium carbonate. Sedatives and hypnotics are frequently used in psychiatry but are commonly in other specialty areas as well and will not be discussed here. Stimulant drugs are prescribed occasionally, but many experts doubt that their effectiveness outweighs the potential for abuse

of these medications. The potential for abuse of the last two groups
of drugs os covered in Chapter 10.

Antipsychotic drugs. Medications was introduced as a treatment
for psychotic behavior in the early 1950s.

Many of the side effects are probably related to the mechanism of
action of these drugs, which is not yet completely understood. It is
suspected that there is probably an interference with dopamine re-
ception or synthesis at the neural synapse. This hypothesis would
also lead to the suspicion that an excess of dopamine contributes to
psychotic behavior, but his is as yet unproved.

There are implications for nursing care related to the side effects
of antipsychotic medications. The nurse should be aware of the most
common side effects and be prepared to teach the patient about them
when they occur. Most side effects are uncomfortable but not dangerous. Following is a summary of those which appear most frequently and the appropriate nursing care:

1. Oversedation. Patients usually feel groggy when they begin to
take antipsychotic medication This ride effect tends to diminish after
the patent taken the medication for a time. It can also be minimized
by giving the whole daily dose of medicine at bedtime, since the
sedating effect does not, last as long as the antipsychotic effect.' If a
patent\ is very upset by the drowsiness. The qualified nurse could
suggest altering the dosage schedule to the physician. It can also be
helpful to explain the side effects to the patient and offer the hope
that it will decrease time.

2. Extrapyramidal effects. Extrapyramidal side effects may produce behaviors similar to those observed in persons with Parkinson's
disease, such a fine tremors, pill-rolling tremor of the fingers drool-
ing, and the characteristic petit pas gain. Related side effects that
occur suddenly and are frightening to the patient are the dystonic
reactions and the oculogyric crisis. The former is a sudden spasm of
the muscles of the face and neck genera; IN, pulling the jaw to one
side and twisting the neck. The latter consists of the eyes
uncontrollably rolling back into the head. Both of these condition,

are generally relieved immediately by intramuscular injection of diphenhydramine hydrochloride (Benadryl) 50 mg, or benztropine mesylate (Cogent 2 mg). A great deal of reassurance is also necessary. Long-term preventive treatment may include change to a different antipsychotic' medications or the addition of an oral antiparkinsonian drug, such as hyxyphenidyl hydrochloride (Artane), procychide hydrochloride (Kemadrin), or benztropine mesylade. There is, however, growing concern about these latter medications over an extended period of time because of the potential for toxic effects, including confusion, dry mouth, blurred vision, or possibly bowel or bladder paralysis. The trend is to use them briefly to deal with parkinsonian side effects but to then discontinue them. It has been found that dystonic reactions tend not to recur after the patient has been taking medications for a time. Any remaining parkinsonian symptoms may be less disturbing to the patient than the side effects of the drugs taken to alleviate them. Another related side effect is aksthisia, or restlessness. This is usually dealt with by substituting another antipsychotic drug.

Tardive dyskinesia is a complication of antipsychotic medication that has recently received much publicity. It is characterized by grimacing moveiemtn of the face, tongue, lips and jaw, uncontrollable choreiform or athetoid movements of the arms, fingers, ankles, or toes; ad tonic contractions of neck and back muscles. This complications usually occurs after high doses of medications have been taken for many years. It has also been irreversible once it occurs, even if the medication is discontinued. All of this Jim has experienced and almost dies four times. One approach that has been taken in an attempt to prevent this problem is the use of "drug holidays," which are scheduled periods of time when the patent takes no medications.

3. Anticholinergic effects. The anticholinergic effect of the antipsychotic drugs influences functioning of the autonomic nervous system and results in a number of side effects, for the most part uncomfortable but not dangerous. One effect that could be serious is orthostatic hypotension. This occurs with particular frequency in the elderly and may require change in medication. The nurse should warn these patients against sudden changes in position and check sitting and standing blood pressure when medications are being introduced. Dry mucous membranes are annoying. Sucking on glycerine-based cough drops sometimes helps the mouth feel moist. Constipation may occur. The nurse should chart bowel movements and offer a laxative as necessary to prevent fecal impaction.

4. Endocrine effects. These may include gynercomastia, lactation, menstrual irregularities, increased libido in women and impotence in ne Patients may be concerned and embarrassed these problems. The nurse can help by providing explanations and reassurance.

5. Allergic reactions. Rashes occasionally with antipsychotic medications and should evaluated by the physician. Usually the medicine is changed and the rash is treated with topic or systemic medication Cholestratic jaundice infrequently and requires discontinuation of medication. Liver function tests should be a periodically or if a patient shows any evidence jaundice .

 6. *Serious blood dyscrasias.* These are rare serious. The nurse should be aware that this occur and report any indication of this complication

7. Photosensitivity. This side effect is particularly associated with chlorpromazine. Patients take this medication should be warned against exposure to direct sunlight and informed about the us sunscreening creams.

The other major problem related to the nurse care of patients who are taking antipsychotic medications cations is that of nonadherence to the treatment plan. Patients need careful explanations about medication schedule and encouragement to medicine regularly. Suspicious patients may continue with medicine at home. Other pat, may stop taking medicine because they feel be In both cases relapse frequently occurs. Some adherent patients are given their antipsychotic medication by depot injection rather than Of Fluphenazine enanthate or decanoate may be given intramuscularly every ten days to three week pending, en the patient's response. Medications usually started orally to evaluate the patient action to it before the injections are started . Nurses must do the same teaching about possible side effects and the necessity for medicine that the with patients who take oral drugs.

Involuntary admission commitment

In the late 1940s the World Health Organization reported that - almost 90% of admissions to state mental hospitals in the United States were involuntary commitments. Conversely, only little more than 10% were voluntary. The trend has definitely shifted to more voluntary admissions. In 1963, 30% were voluntary, and by 1971 nearly half' of all admissions to psychiatric hospitals were initiated by the patient himself If. 3 This trend is due to the greater variety of admission statuses and more stringent limitations placed on the use of involuntary commitment. This is still in striking contrast to England, however, where over 89% of the patients are admitted voluntarily.

Involuntary commitment does not always imply compulsion. It means that the request for hospitalization did not originate with the patient and may signify that either it was actively opposed by him or signify that either it was actively opposed by him or as indecisive and did not resist. The criteria for commitment vary among states and reflect the confusion present in the medical, social, and legal arenas of society. Most laws justify commitment of the mentally ill on three grounds: dangerous to others, dangerous to self, and need for treatment. The important element appears to be whether the person can function in a reasonable manner in the outside world without becoming an undue burden on his family or the community. The vagueness of the criteria is reflected in the patients committed to psychiatric hospitals. Those suffering from psychoses account for less than half of all admissions, and the aged, the neurotic, and others account for less than half of all admissions, and the aged, the neurotic, and others account for the majority.

State laws on commitment vary, but they attempt to protect the individual who is not mentally ill from being detained in a psychiatric hospital against his will for political, economic, family, Or other nonmedical reasons. Certain procedural elements of the commitment

process are common. Action is begun with a sworn petition by a
relative friend, public official, physician, or any interested citizen
stating the person is mentally ill and is it, need of treatment. Some
states allow only specific individuals to file such a petition. An examination of the patient's mental status is then completed by one or
two physicals. Some state require at leas one of the physicians to be
a psychiatrist.

The decision as to whether the patient requires,, hospitalization is
then made. Precisely who makes, this decision determines the nature
of the commitment. Medical certification means a specified number
of appointed physicians make the decision. This power to certify is
given to all physicians and not limited to psychiatrists. Court or judicial commitment is decided on by a judge or jury in a formal bearing.

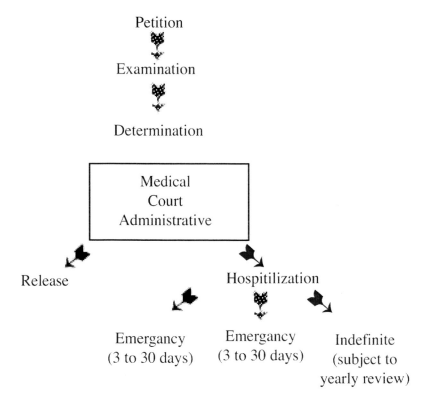

Fig 12-1: Diagrammatical model of the involuntary commitment process

In this case the court is required to notify the e patient so that be can retain legal counsel to prepare for the hearing if he desires to contest it. A jury trial is not mandatory in most states but can be requested by the patient. Most states recognize the right of the patient to have legal counsel, but only Out half actually appoint a lawyer for the patient he does not have one. Administrative commitment determined by a special tribunal of hearing officer. The Fourteenth Amendment to the United States Constitution protects citizens against infringements on liberty without "due process of the law." Because of this, medical certification is used infrequently and primarily in emergency situations, an administrative commitment is subject to judicial review.

If the individual is determined to be in need of treatment, the final step of the commitment process will occurs and he is hospitalized. This may be for serving lengths of time depending on the needs of the patient. Fig. 12-1 presents a diagrammatic model of the involuntary commitment process. It identifies three types of hospitalization: emergency, temporary, and indefinite.

Emergency hospitalization. Almost all states have provisions for emergency commitment for patients, rho are acutely ill. The goals for the commitment it short-term and it is primarily intended as a means of controlling an immediate threat to self or others. In those states tracking such a law the acutely ill individual is often taken into custody by the police and kept in jail on a disorderly conduct charge, which is a criminal charge. Such a practice is inappropriate and frequently detrimental to the mental status of the patient.

To obtain an emergency commitment the patient's family, a physician or someone designated by the state must file a petition that includes a supporting report by a psychiatrist. It is then reviewed by a judge or hospital official and hospitalization is provided. Most state laws limit the time, the person can be detained under emergency commitment to From three to thirty days. Emergency hospitalization allows for detainment in a psychiatric hospital only until proper legal steps are taken to provide for additional hospitalization.

Temporary or observational hospitalization. This type of

commitment is primarily used for the purpose pose of diagnosis
and short-term therapy and does not require an emergency situation,
as does the emergency hospitalization. Again, the commitment is for
a specified period of time, but in this case it ranges from two to six
months. The commitment process is similar to that just described.
Some states require a court order for -all temporary commitments,
whereas others require one only if the person protests the hospitalization. If at the end of the stipulated period of time the patient is still
not ready for discharge, a petition can be filed for an indefinite commitment.

Indefinite hospitalization (formal commitment) A formal commitment provides for the hospitalization of a patient for an indetermi-
nate amount of time or until he is ready for discharge. The process is
usually that of a court commitment. Patients in public or state mental
hospitals more frequently have indefinite commitments than patients
in private hospitals. Even when committed, these patients maintain
their right to consult a lawyer at any time and to request a court hearing to determine if additional hospitalization is necessary. The hospital ultimately discharges the patient, however, and a court order is
not necessary to do this.

Commitment dilemma

In seventeen states involuntary commitment assumes incompetency and is accompanied by the patient's loss of his civil rights. He
is restricted in his ability to make contracts, vote, drive, obtain a
professional license, serve on a jury, marry, or enter into civil litiga-
tion. In addition, the patient must suffer the stigma attached to the
label "committed" in all his future activities. Because of the large
numbers of people affected by involuntary commitment and the loss
of personal rights that it entails, it becomes a matter of great legal,
moral, social, and psychiatric significance. In the practice of general
medicine there is no equivalent divestment of individual rights except for rare cases of mandated quarantine for carriers of some potentially epidemic diseases.

The question may be asked "How disturbed or ill does one need to be to merit commitment as insane?" A psychotic state is not a necessary or sufficient cause for commitment, as evident in the number of elderly, addicted, and neurotic patients hospitalized as well as the many psychotic individuals who remain at liberty. Perhaps a person's dangerousness to himself or others is a more pertinent consideration. Certainly psychiatric professionals consider hospitalization in this instance as a humanitarian gesture and as a protection of the individual and society. "Dangerousness," however, is an undefined, unspecified term.

It is interesting to note that people who are mentally health,.., and dangerous have their freedom guarded by the courts so that after a prison sentence is served.. the individual is automatically released and can no longer be retained. However, someone who is mentally ill and dangerous can be confined indefinitely. Ennis states: "Of all the identifiably dangerous groups in society, only the mentally ill are singled out for preventive detention and . . . they are probably the least dangerous as a group. Why should society confine a person if he is dangerous and mentally ill but not if he is dangerous and sane?" To support his suggestion that the mentally ill are probably less dangerous than the mentally healthy, he cites a five-year study of 5000 patients discharged from a state mental hospital in New York. The results showed that their arrest rate was one-twelfth that of the general population. The idea of preventive detention does not exist in most areas of the law where the ability to predict an action does not confer the right to control the ion in advance. Only illegal acts result in a prolonged loss of liberty for most citizens. Except the mentally ill.

Another aspect of this dilemma also revolves around this idea of dangerousness. Even if some mentally ill individuals are potentially dangerous, it has not been proved that psychiatrists are good predictors of future violence. Frequently psychiatrists over-predict the patient's potential for dangerous acts and the extent of his illness. Oran believes this is because of the medical training of the psychiatrist, which has taught him that underdiagnosis is more harmful than overdiagnosis.

For some time now I have maintained that commitment is, the detention of persons in mental institutions against their will is a form of imprisonment; such deprivation of liberty is contrary to the moral principles embodied in the Declaration of Independence '" Constitution of the United States: and that it is a is violation of contemporary concepts of fundamental human rights. The practice of sane men incarcerating insane fellow men in 'mental hospitals" can be ,pared to that of white men enslaving black men. In fact, I consider commitment a crime against humanity

Whether to take a stand for or against commitment is an issue each nurse must resolve for herself. What should be done if the nonconformist does wish to change his behavior" Does he maintain freedom to choose even if his thinking appears to be irrational or divergent from the norm? Does the divergent of mutuality exclude coercion? Can social concept of interests be served by a means less restrictive than total confinement, such as outpatient therapy? Every nurse should assume the responsibility for reviewing the commitment procedures in her state and work for legislative amendments that would facilitate the necessary reforms.

The commitment dilemma therefore exposes present practices and opens areas of controversy for the future The present mental hospital has been described as a jail, a hospital, a poorhouse, and a home for the elderly. It protects, treats, feeds, maintains, and houses socially incompetent individuals who are often feared by society When they are discharged from the hospital, they are frequently left without alternatives and come to the attention of law enforcement agencies or welfare offices. Local communities deny the problem by resisting the establishment of halfway houses or sheltered homes in their neighborhood. Third-party insurance seldom covers extended outpatient psychiatric care. In today's mobile and impersonal society, family and friends are often unwilling or unable to care For the newly released patient, who many end up in a dismal run-down hotel or boarding house with nothing to do but watch television and wander the streets.

These issues need to be addressed by psychiatric nurses, patients. And citizens across the country The value of commitment, the goals of hospitalization the quality of life, and the rights of patients must be closely aligned and resolved through the judicial, the legislative, and the medical systems.

Discharge

A patient who voluntarily admits himself into the hospital can be discharged by the staff when he has received "maximum benefit" from the treatment or he may initiate his own discharge request. Most states require that he give written notice of his desire for discharge and some hospitals will also request he sign a form that states he is leaving against media advice." These forms then become part of his permanent record.

Listed on the next page are the Rights of A client that is or has been "classified" as mentally ill, nuts, crazy, weird, strange (unique would be too complimentary-) or simply different from the "norm"- (societies accepted rules to breathe) in that ....they are either: Non-hypocritical-Brave enough to deviate periodically and laugh at the hilarious-or they are truthful enough be or not to be", (then of course comes the question maybe, possibly, they are close enough to God to hear the words He speaks to them ... therefore, they are just -fortunate enough now to love the Church, but know the need to enter the Chambers of Solitude and gossip, etc. is not for the expurgation of weekly sins ... and under the Oak tree with God's-so much more successful to purify and start over: ..... Another important "unique" gift-now sometimes classified as a sign of mental illness from process of Eliminations in behavior therapy is the most precious and misused word in the vocabulary for all mankind Love! Its only true meaning as it was first defined is in Corinthians, and is truly as hard to comprehend by mortals-I guess-as the virgin-birth Nevertheless-it has been adopted-and attempted to dwell by, and ironic. Ironically as it seems, really felt by some people. This is where I feel, personally. Jim, (as one of my very best friends) has fallen short of acceptance in behavior lately and it is because of the proven physical and mental anguish, turmoil, oil, strife, depression, demoralization, ? physical contact, denial to the Actional facts, and lied to with the obvious since Day 1. This is the cause of destructional disaster for making-You doubt me. Ask God.

Allowing for great variation among states, patents presently have the following rights:

- Right to communicate with people outside the hospital through correspondence, telephone, and personal visits Right to keep clothing and personal effects with them in the hospital
- Right to religious freedom
- Right to be employed if possible
- Right to manage and dispose of property Right to ex ecute wills
- Right to enter into contractual relationships Right to make purchases
- Right to education
- Right to habeas corpus
- Right to independent psychiatric examination Right to civil service status
- Right to retain licenses, privileges, or permits estab lished by law, such as a driver's or professional license
- Right to sue or be sued.
- Right to marry and divorce
- Right not to be subject to unnecessary mechanical re straints
- Right to periodic review of status Right to legal repre sentation
- Right to privacy
- Right of informed consent Right to treatment
- Right to treatment in the least restrictive setting

Some of these rights merit exploration in greater detail.

Right to communicate with people outside the hospital. This right entails the freedom of the patient to visit and hold telephone conversations in privacy and send unopened letters to anyone of his choice, including judges, lawyers, families, and staff. On occasions hospital staff have intercepted letters presumed to be threatening or abusive and disposed of them. In states where this is not illegal, such activity raises the moral question of individual freedom versus the good of the community.

Right to keep personal effects. This establishes the right of the patient to bring clothing and personal items with him to the hospital, taking into consideration the amount of space available for storage of them. It does not make the hospital responsible for their safety. Valuable items should preferably be left at home. If the patient brings something of value to the hospital, the staff should place it in the hospital safe or make other appropriate provisions for its safekeeping.

Right to be employed if possible. This includes the right to work whenever possible and the right to be compensated for it, including payment for work-therapy programs within the hospital. Ivoluntary servitude or work without pay within institutions is on the decline because courts have held that the Thirteenth Amendment, which abolished slavery, also applies to psychiatric patients. The consequence of these decisions is that mental institutions cannot force patients to work, either by punishing them or by making privileges or discharge dependent on work. If patients choose to work, they must be assigned jobs on documented therapeutic grounds and they must be paid the minimum wage.

The Department of Labor is notifying all institutions that if they fail to pay patient workers, they are violating the law. The ultimate effect of this move is not yet known. Some professionals fear that the money to pay patients will come out of treatment funds and that the patients will fare worse in the end. Others fear that hospitals will hire regular labor and leave the patients with nothing to do. Some argue that institutions will charge pateints for room and board and recover much of the money. A further fear raised is that if the Department of Labor enforces the law and if institutions comply, they may be forced to close because of lack of funds.

Right to execute wills. A person's competency to make a will is known as testamentary capacity. He can make a valid will if he (1) knows that he is making a will; (2) knows the nature and extent of his property, and (3) knows who his friends and relatives are and what the relationships mean. Each of these criteria must be met for the will to be considered valid. This means he must not be mentally confused at the time he signed his will. It does not imply that he must have the exact details of his property holdings or specific bank account figures. But he cannot attempt to give away more than be possesses. Furthermore, the law requires that he know who his relatives are but does not require him to bequeath anything to them.

The fact that a patient is committed or is diagnosed as psychotic does not immediately invalidate his will. The will is valid if it was made during a lucid period and the patient met the three criteria. The problem most debated in determining testamentary capacity is the delusional patient, particularly if the delusional thinking could alter the outcome of the will. The important question in this regard is whether the false belief or delusion caused the person to dispose of his property, in a different way than he would have otherwise

Two or three persons must witness the will by watching the person as he signs it and each other as they sign it. It is necessary therefore that they A be together at this time. At a later time a nurse may be summoned into court to give testimony on the condition of the person at the time he drew up his will. The nurse should testify relative to the three criteria as well as report pertinent observations, recall information as accurately as possible, and express herself concisely and objectively. Hospital charts may also be used in the court proceedings, and the nurse's notes relative to the patient's behavior and mental status may provide additional information.

Right to enter into contractual relationships. Contracts are considered valid by the court if the person understands the circumstances involved in the contract and the natural consequences of it. Once again, a psychiatric illness does not invalidate a contract, although the nature of the contract and degree of judgment needed to understand it would be influencing factors.

Incompetency. An issue related to this right is the one of mental incompetency. Every adult is assumed to be mentally competent and possess the mental abiltiy to carry out his affairs. To prove otherwise requires a special court bearing to declare him "incompetent." This is a legal term without a preprecise medical meaning. To prove that ail individual is incompetent it must be shown that (1) he has mental disorder, (2) this disorder causes a defect judgment, and (3) this defect makes him incapable of handling his own affairs. All three elements be present. and the exact diagnostic label is lot important in this regard. If a person is declared competent, a legal guardian will be appointed by the court to manage the patient's estate. This frequently is a family member, friend, or bank executive. Incompetency rulings are most often filed for persons with senile dementia, cerebral arteriosclerosis, chronic schizophrenia, and mental retardation.

The trend in legislation is to separate the concepts of incompetency and involuntary committment since the reasons for each are esentially different. Incompetency arises from society's desire to safeguard a person's assets from his own inability to understand and transact business. Involunatry committments are usually initiated to protect the patient from himself (in the case of suicide), protect others from the patient (in the case of homicide), and administer treatment. However, many states still consider the two equivalent, and the policies and procedures of the hospital may impose the incompetent status on the patient.

As a result of an incompetency ruling, the person cannot vote, marry, drive, or make contracts. A release from the hospital is not necessarily an automatic restoration to competency. Rather. another court bearing is required to reverse the previous ruling and declare the individual competent and allow him to once again manage his own affair

Right to education. This right is being exercise by many parents on behalf of their emotionally ill or mentally retarded children. Everyone is guarantee this right under the constitution, although many states have not made provisions for the adequate education of all groups of citizens and are now being required to do so.

Right to habeas corpus. Habeas corpus is an important right the person retains in all states even if he has been involuntarily admitted to the hospital. It originated in English Common Law and is provided for in the Constitution of the United States. The object of the writ is the speedy release of any idividual who claims he is being deprived of his liberty and detained illegally. A committed patient may file such a writ at any time on the grounds that he is sane and eligible for release. The hearing takes place in a court of law where those people who serve to restrain the patient must defend their actions. A jury is sometimes impaneled to determine the sanity if the patient. A determination is then made, and if the court finds the patient to be sane, he is discharged from the hospital.

Right to independent psychiatric examination. Under the Emergency Admission Statute the patient has the right to demand a psychiatric examination by a physician of his own choice. If this physician determines that he is not mentally ill, the patient must be released.

Right to marry and divorce. Since marriage is a formal contract, the same general criteria for validity apply that is, the marriage is considered valid if the idiividaul understands the nature of the marriage relationship and the duties and obligations it entails. The crucial element is his mental capacity at the time of the marriage, not before it or after it. In general, courts are reluctant to declare a marriage void. Many states have laws forbidding the marriage of mentally ill persons. This is based on the notion that mental illness, whether genetically or environmentally induced, often runs in families. Thus the primary objective of such laws is to prevent the procreation of children who might be mentally ill. In these cases the law is not based on any scientific evidence of the inheritability of mental illness.

In most states psychiatric illness is not in itself grounds for divorce. However, some states will grant divorces if the mentally ill spouse has been committed to a hospital for a certain number of years, unsually three to five. It is sometimes also necessary to specify that the spouse is "incurably insane." psychiatric professionals are hesitant to make such a determination.

Right to privacy. The right to privacy implies the right of the individual to keep some information about himself completely secret from others. Confidentially involves the disclosure of certain information mation to another person, but this is limited to specifically authorized individuals. It is the responsibility of every psychiatric professional to safeguard a patient's right to confidentiality in all aspects of psychiatric treatment, including even the knowledge that a person is in therapy or in a hospital. Revealing such information might damage a person's reputation or hamper his ability to obtain a job. This was most dramatically evident when Senator Eagleton was running as a vice-presidential candidate in the 1972 presidential election. The issue of confidentiality is becoming increasingly important, since various agencies demand information about a patient's history, diagnosis, treatment, and prognosis and sophisticated methods for obtaining information (such as wiretapping and computer banks) have been developed. These threaten the individual's right to privacy. The clinician is free from legal responsibility if information is released with the patient's written and signed request. As a rule it is best to reveal as little information as possible and discuss with the patient what the material will be.

The concept of confidentiality builds on the element of trust necessary in a patient/therapist relationship. The patient places himself in the care of others and reveals vulnerable aspects of his personal life. In return he expects high-quality care and the safeguard of his interests. Thus the patient/therapist relationship is an intimate one and demands trust, loyalty, and the maintenance of privacy.

The phrase *privileged communication* is a legal one and applies only in court-related preceedings. It includes communications between husband and wife, attorney and client, and clergyman and church member. The right to reveal information belongs to the person who spoke, and the listener cannot disclose the information unless the speaker gives permission. This privilege exists for the protection of the patient. Privileged communication between other professionals and a patient exists only if a law specifically establishes it. Thirty-eight states curretly recognize privileged

communication between physicians and patients, twelve do not. Four
states have laws providing for privileged communication between
nurses and patients, including Arkansas, New York. New Mexico.
and South Dakota. All the other states do not, and a nurse would be
required to reveal what the patient said to her in a court of law. In
general, however, it is rare that a nurse is called into court to divulge
information of this kind.

Most hospitals keep psychiatric records separately and provide
that they are less accessible than medical records. They are viewed
by the law and psychiatric profession to he more sensitive than general medical records. Psychiatrists, for the most part, retain the right
to decide if they should release medical information to the patient,
and in some states patients are barred from viewing them at all. A
hospital chart can be summoned into court, however, and anything
that is written in it can be used in a lawsuit. Privileged communication does not apply to hospital charts, and nursing notes should be
written carefully in all cases. Furthermore, it is a general rule that
only those persons involved in a patient's rare may read his chart.
This includes physicians, nurses, aides, students, and others directly
involved in the treatment process.

Right to informed consent. Informed consent includes the disclosure by a physician of a certain amount of information to the patient
about the proposed treatment and the attainment of the patient's consent, which must be competent, understanding, and voluntary. The
physician must explain the special treatment, its possible complications, and its risks. The patient must be capable of giving consent
and not be a minor or judged incompetent or insane by the court.
Failure to obtain consent may be the basis for lawsuits of "assault
and battery" or negligence.

Psychiatric outpatients usually express their consent by their will-
ingness to come for treatment, and only unusual treatments such as
experimental drugs or electroconvulsive therapy require specific
written consent. Informally admitted and voluntary patients usually
sign a paper on admission consenting to psychiatric treatment, which
includes milieu therapy, chemotherapy, psychotherapy, and

occupational therapy. Unusual treatments again need special permission. In the care of the involuntarily admitted patient, the commitment procedure gives the hospital the right to treat the patient.

Consent forms usually require the signature patient, a family member, and two persons who witnessed their signing it. Nurses are frequetnly called on in this regard. It then becomes a part the patient's permanent hospital record.

Right to treatment. The concept of the right treatment is a relatively recent development. In 1960 Birnbaum, a graduate student in both medicine and law, wrote, "there does not appear to have been any significant and realistic consideration given, from a legal viewpoint, to the problem of whether or not the institutionalized mentally ill person receives adequate medical treatment so that be may regain his health, and therefore his liberty as soon as possible. " This cause received its impetus with a 1966 case in the District of Columbia (Rouse v. Vameron). The court held that mental patients committed by criminal courts had the right to adequate treatment. Furthermore, it said that confinement without treatment was tantamount to incarceration and thus transformed the hospital into a penitentiary. It affirmed that the purpose of involuntary hospitalization was treatment. not punishment and if this treatment was not provided, the patient could be transferred, released. or even awarded damages for his period of confinement. The court clarified that the hospital did not need to show that the treatment would improve or cure the patient but only that there was a true attempt to do so.

This right to treatment was extended in 1972 to a mentally ill and mentally retarded persons who were involuntarily hospitalized in a case in Alabama (Wyatt v. Stickney). The court stated: "To deprive any citizen of his or her liberty upon the altruistic theory that the confinement is for humane therapeutic tic reasons and then fail to provide adequate treatment violates the very fundamentals of due process." It further defined criteria for adequate treatment in three areas: (1) a humane psychological and physical environment, (2) a qualified staff with a sufficient number of members to administer adequate treatment, and (3) individualized treatment plans. The keystone of the Wyatt decision is the requirement that an individualized treatment plan be for mulated.

There are no existing solutions to these complex issues, but they are of concern to nurses who are frequently responsible for delivering prescribed treatment modalities such as medications.

At this time nurses should make their judgments on a case-by-case basis. The Task Force on Behavior Therapy has examined the issue of coerced treatment and suggested three criteria that may justify it :

1. The patient must be judged to be dangerous to himself or others.

2. It must be believed by those administering treatment that it has a reasonable chance to benefit the patient and those related to him.

3. The patient must be judged to be incompetent to evaluate the necessity of the treatment.

They stress that even if these three conditions are met, the patient should not be deceived. He should be informed as to what will be done to him, the reasons for it, and its probable effects.

Future court decisions will certainly explore the many aspects of this issue. Peck indicates possible outcomes:

> The right-to-treatment movement . . . will undoubtedly do away with some of the injustices and deplorable conditions that have resulted in support for the right to refuse treatment and involuntary hospitalization. The end result might be more humane hospitals and treatment, which would lessen the impact of this movement. On-the other hand, the right to treatment will probably also tend to mark make hospitals froce their treatment, out of fear of being sued on persons who were previously ignored. This in turn might result in an increase maintaining the right to refuse treatment

Right to treatment in the least restrictive setting. The right to treatment in the least restrictive setting is closely related to the right to adequate treatment. It refers to the goal of evaluating the specific needs of each patient and maintaining the greatest amount of personal freedom, autonomy, dignity, and integrity in determining the treatment or services he is to receive. This right applies to both community and noncom muity-based programs. Greater consideration of this right might well limit some of the controversial surrounding the commitment dilemma and the right to refuse treatment.

Nursing's role in patients' rights

The National League for Nursing, in 1977 issued a statement on the nurse's role in patients' rights. Respect and concern for patients and assurance of competent care were identified as basic rights, along with patients receiving the information they need to understand their illness and make decisions about their care. The League urged nurses to directly involve themselves in assuring the human and legal riots of patients.

Many of the patients' rights identified by the League include those previously mentioned. They also list the following rights*:
- Right to health care that is accessible and that meets professional standards. regardless of the setting.
- Right to courteous and individualized health care that is equitable, humane, and given without discrimination as to race, color, creed, sex. national origin, source of payment, or ethical or political beliefs.
- Right to information about their diagnosis prognosis, and treatment, including laternatives to care and risks involved.
- Right to information about the qualifications. names and titles of personel responsible for providing their health care.
- Right to refuse ovservation by those not directly involed
- in their care.
- Right to coordination and continuity of health care.
- Right to information on the charges for services including eluding the right to challenge these.

* National League for Nursing Nursing's role in patient's rights. New York. 1977.
the League. Used with permission.

• Above all,the right to be fully informed-as to a]! the rights
in all health care settings.

LITIGATION AND PSYCHIATRIC NURSING

All psychiatric professionals have legally defines duties of care
and are responsible for their own work. If these duties are violated,
malpractice exist. Malpractice involves the failure of profession person to give the kind of proper and complete care that is given by
members of his profession the community resulting in harm to the
patient. Most malpractice claims are filed under the law of negligent
tort. A tort is a civil wrong for which the injured party is entitled to
compensation. Because under the law, everyone is responsible for
his own torts, each nurse can be held responsible in malpractice practice claims. Under the law of negligent tort the plaintiff must prove
the following:
1. A legal duty of care existed.
2. the nurse perfromed the duty negligently.
3. Damages were suffered by the plaintiff as a result.
4. The damages were substanital.

Emotions and behavior

OBJECTIVES
• *To understand the meaning of emotion.*
• *To understand the types of emotion commonly experienced by
everyone.*
• *To become increasingly aware of emotions as influences on
behavior.*

MEANING OF EMOTIONS
Emotions are those inner feelings which all of us have. They are
patterns of response to life situations, varying in type and intensity

according to the experience of the moment. Many different terms are used tp describe emotions. Some of these terms describe the type of feeling; other terms imply the intensity of the feeling.

Emotions are neither good nor bad. We all experience these iner feelings according to what is happening to us and how we preceive that event. To think of any emotion as "good" or "bad" in a moral sense is pointless, just as it would be pointless to think of being hungry as "good" or "bad." Both the positive and the negative emotions are natural reactions to life experiences. The effests of the negative emotions are unpleasant, but they have a definite purpose as natural reactions to displeasing or threatening experiences.

IMPORTANCE OF EMOTIONS

Emotions have physical, mental and spiritual effects. Indirectly they determine the amount of satisfaction one gets from life, the degree of success in solving life problems, and the satisfaction found in relations with other people. We must learn to use our emotions;

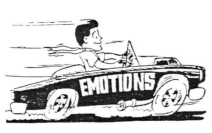
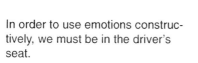

In order to use emotions constructively, we must be in the driver's seat.

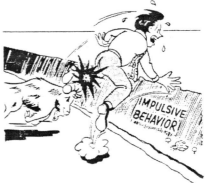

Repressed emotions can erupt suddenly and propel an individual into undesirable behavior.

otherwise, we allow emotions to exert too influence on our behavior. The person who is competent in dealing with his life problems has learned to use his emotions constructively. They serve his purposes and are expressed in socially acceptable ways. Unless emotions are used effectively and Oven adequate expression, they are likely to erupt suddenly and uncontrollably in undesirable behavior.

Do you wonder whether emotions can be this important? Consider for a moment. Can you think clearly when you are angry? Do you burst into tears, run away from the situation, throw things, or swear? Or do you hold your anger in and pretend that you are perfectly calm? Can you think clearly when you are extremely unhappy? Do you feel hatred or bitterness toard the cause of your unhappiness! How do you feel physically energetic or listless?

If you have mentally reviewed some past experiences which aroused anger, fear, or sorrow, then you probably agree that emotions do have physical and mental effects.

Physical Effects

Emotions influence physical functioning, with particular effect on the autonomic nervous system. The autonomic nervous system. in turn. influences the functioning of internal organs. Through this indirect influence, the emotional state can stimulate certain organs and inhibit the activity of others. The balance of body chemicals affected by strong emotional states: this effect is extreme but of short duration.

In states of moderate emotional arousal such as chronic anxiety, this effect is less extreme, but it keeps the internal processes in a state of "semi-emergency alert." Over a period of time, this long-term physiological situation can lead to actual physical changes, such as ulcers.

Formation of Emotional Patterns

Emotional arousal is closely related to everything we have already discussed about behavior. Patterns are learned through experience and according to the satisfaction or distress resulting from life experiences. Each person's capacity to feel different emotions may be hereditary: newborn infants show marked differences in their responses to distress. In spite of possible hereditary, differences, the great differences in adult emotional responses are probably due mostly to learning. Environment determines what some of these learings will be. The social enviornment the people of a baby's world determine to a great degree whether the baby's experiences are pleasing or distressing. Later in life the balance of successes and failures in daily living have great influence on emotional patterns. Throughout life the reactions of other people to one's expressions of emotion influence future expressions of emotion.

Emotions, then, do not lend themselves to a simple definition. Rather, they must be considered within the framework of other influences on behavior: heredity, environment, basic needs, life experiences, and interaction with other people.

THE POSITIVE EMOTIONS

Happiness

The positive emotions might be thought of as those which make us feel good. Happiness is a general sense of well-being. This emotion might be described as joy or elation if the felling of happiness is strong. If the feeling is less intense, it might be described as pleasure or satisfaction. Each of these terms implies lies not only the specific emotion but also the intensity.

Love

Love is an important positive emotion. Strong feelings of warmth for another person might be thought of as love, with milder feelings of the same type being termed friendliness. Affection implies a feeling less intense than love, but stronger than friendliness. Love implies caring about someone else, being concerned enough to help and understand, and respect the person loved. Love in this sense affects the relationship we have with others of both sexes. The capacity of a person to feel love influences that person's outlook on life and his attitudes toward mankind in general. The ability to love and to receive love is important in -all of living. It is learned or not teamed early in life and modified by life experiences.

Kinds of Love

There are many kinds of love: the love of a mother for her child; the child's love, at first self-centered and then extended to others; love for one's playmates; love for material things associated with pleasant memories; love for friends with whom life experiences have been shared; love for unfortunate ones wherever they might be; love for a patient and his family, all struggling with their stressful situation. Sexual love should involve both self-love and selfless love, the desire for oneness with the loved one including a desire to please which exceeds the desire to be pleased Spiritual love is different still and varies according to one's concept of the Divinity. Needless to say, each kind of love is expressed in its own way. Newspaper accounts of some family's misfortune often result in a flood of contributions from strangers, illustrating the capacity of many people to love those who are less fortunate than themselves.

Love for Self and Others

Love, you may be surprised to learn, must begin with love of self. The baby's love is egocentric, that is, self-centered; baby love is closely tied in with receiving satisfaction from others. During childhood, one gradually teams to love others, but love of self tends to dominate throughout childhood. gradually, the child teams to extend love to others. This learning prepares for the development of such traits as generosity and courtesy, as opposed to "good manners." As development proceeds, the ability to love others begins to dominate self-love. People who do not have self-love those whose selfconcept is that of an unworthy I person, and those who have strong fellings of guilt. often have difficulty in establishing Satisfying relations with other people. This relationship between self-love and love of others will become clearer as we explore adjustment and other aspects of interpersonal relations.

NEGATIVE EMOTIONS

The negative emotions are those which make us feel uncomfortable. The intensity of each of these emotions can range from a mild state to a very strong one, with various possible grandations of feeling in between these two extremes. The effects on the individual may be a vague restlessness, a feeling of dissatisfaction, or a state of intense agitation.

Fear and Anger

Anger is an emotion aroused by obstacles, threat, or otherwise offensive situations. It is usually directed at a specific object or person, but it can be generalized, as anger at the world in general or at Society. Hate may be thought of as intense anger felt toward a specific person or persons, though hate often includes an element of fear. Annoyance is used to describe a mild form of anger. Rage describes intense anger and often implies expression of the anger through violent physical activity.

Fear is an emotion aroused primarily by threat. The threat may be related to physical harm or it may be related to one's sense of security. Fear of physical harm is usually of short duration; the danger passes or the person is able to escape the dangerous situation. Fear of loss of a job, loss of money or other property, or loss of loved ones may continue for a long period. When such fear is chronic, it is known as anxiety. Apprehension is used to describe mild fear, while I terror and panic describe intense fear.

Fear and anger cause the body to mobilize for action for fighting or fleeing a threatening situation. The body response is an outpouring of adrenalin, which increases the flow of blood through the body, raises the rate of respiration, and simulates muscle tone. The body under these circumstances is literally mobilized for action. If physical activity does not occur, this readiness for action may be released through "the shakes."

Then the rational approach is to withdraw from that situation. If similar unhappy experiences occur in the new setting, then probably a close took at oneself is indicated. Perhaps the source of the problem is self rather than others.

Withdrawal in the sense of placing a barrier between oneself and others — the world, so to speak — is a psychiatric symptom. Poorly adjusted people who show signs of increasing tendencies to withdraw from friends and family are showing signs of a need for professional help. Too often such behavior is allowed to continue for long periods, and the family says, "Oh, he just likes to be by himself."

Some of the defense mechanisms already discussed represent withdrawal to some extent. Daydreaming is withdrawal for a short period of time. Retreat into illness may also be thought of as a type of withdrawal.

DEFENSE MECHANISMS AND ADJUSTMENT

Differences in Perception of Threat

All of us need to use adjustment mechanisms of many types, including defense mechanisms. We all have unhappy experiences. We all have problem situations to face. We all encounter obstacles in our efforts to achieve our goals. We all experience disappointment and failure at intervals. Each of us has a self-concept which we struggle to maintain. When circumstances threaten that self-concept, we tend to become defensive.

A situation threatening to you may not bother your best friend.

Conversely, you may wonder why another situation upsets your friend. Some of us become defensive any time we are criticized. some of us become apprehensive when we are expected to show achievement: some of us become uncomfortable in the presence of an authority figure; some of us are distrustful of strangers. The situation which is threatening, then, is quite personal. It is based co a great extent on the sensitive areas, or psychological scars. resulting from past hurtful experiences.

The Patient

As a health worker, keep in mind chat illness and hospitalization represnet threat to most people. Therefore, you are likely to see many examples of defense mechanisms as you work with patients.

As you become more aware of your tendencies to use defense mechanisms, you should even begin to recognize those you have previously been using unconsciously. This awareness will not come overnight, nor will it come without some effort on your part to study your behavior patterns.

With increasing understanding of yourself and your use of defense mechanisms, you will be ready to modify habits: to eliminate self-deception, to learn to face reality, and to use appropriate behavior in a variety of situations. Through practice in dealing with problems rather than "fleeing" from them, you can improve your skills in solving problems, even those which involve some unpleasantness. As you grow in your ability to live effectively, you Will have less need for defense mechanisms.

SUGGESTED ACTIVITIES

The following topics are suggested for small group discussion:
1. A clinical laboratory worker breaks an expensive piece of equipment and uses one of the following defense mechanisms:
   a. Projection
   b. Withdrawal

c. Rationalization

d. Escape into illness

2. Situations the following people might perceive as threatening:

a. A practical nurse whose supervisor reminds her of her mother. As a child she felt she could never please her mother, for she was criticized frequently.

b. A surgical technician student who is very capable but never did do well in school, especially after he had a teacher who graded very strictly and often told him he was just too lazy to learn.

Adjustments to marriage, parenthood and job responsibilities all involve numerous frustrations. Even after one has learned to function within the various roles of adulthood, frustrations occur in each role periodically. Life does not flow smoothly, and many of the problems it presents are examples of frustration. Competition is characteristic of modern society; a competitor is adways an obstacle or a potential obstacle, whether a coworker, an opponent in sports, or a neighbor with a new car.

COPING WITH FRUSTRATION

There are innumerable ways of dealing with frustration. The most desirable method for handling one particular frustration may be quite inappropriate for handling another. The general approach requires two steps:

• Expect a certain amount of frustration in living and avoid overreacting emotionally or feeling that you have more bad luck than other people.

• Learn to recognize frustration when it occurs and then deal with it effectively, avoiding defensive reactions.

Ineffective Ways of Dealing With Frustration

The defense mechanisms provide a variety of ways to react to frustration, but they usually do not further one's progress toward the desired goal. They merely provide temporary relief from the feelings accompanying the frustration. The person who uses ineffective methods of dealing with frustration may blame someone else or circumstances for his failure, may rationalize, may displace his anger (and or fear), may become openly aggressive or hostile toward the obstacle, or may settle for a lesser goal. As far as effort is concerned, these represent the easy way out, but they do not usually enable, one to reach the desired goal

Effective Ways of Dealing With Frustration

There is no guaranteed way to overcome any and all obstacles. It is necessary to recognize that the negative feelings of the moment are due to frustration, and then attempt to use a rational approach to solve the problem at hand. The following questions can produce answers for realistic planning to overcome the obstacle:
  • Exactly what goal am I trying to reach?

Haldol:
Haldol mixed with lithium has been known to cause brain damage and death. Jim has been exposed to this mixture on four occasions in which he come very close to death each time. Besides, after the first does, his wife gave him it was a known fact that Jim was highly allergic to Haldol. Jim says God saved his live.

SUMMARY

Part of a mentally healthy state is being able to bear certain kinds of painful feelings. This implies not avoiding the genuine painful feeling by using other defensive feelings or not substituting behavior or a though disorder for that feeling. That is not to say that all feelings are normal or that the expression of feeling is always healthy or appropriate, however, bearing certain genuinely painful feelings is often the "healthiest" way to deal with certain conditions.

I know, by close and sincere observations with Jim, that he has truly faced and challenged all the heartaches he has been faced with, (even since I have been working with him.). When he has been "keyed-up" it has always been most understandable and quite normal. He talks about his problems and listens for suggestions...and takes them. This is so true by the fact he so submitted himself totally, last year to everyone's unprofessional gestures for Jim.

I think, personally it is absolutely pathetic, how another person could unblanket the security of a professional man, and his business, and then demand his soul in return. For Jim to stand for what is true and for just himself as a man of reason...I think with all the behaviors I have dealt with, he has been nothing less than a gentleman, a good father and a caring, concerned individual for everyone involved!

CHAPTER XI

IN CONCLUSION: WORDS OF INSPIRATION

Now that you understand the seriousness of your condition, you should be sure and seek (if you don't already have) a good doctor in this field that you can trust your life with.

Now that you have read this book, keep it and buy one for your family, and encourage them to read it, to better understand you.

Please read these closing poems and messages in hopes that they will inspire you as they have inspired me. A manic depressive often needs inspiration from within as well as from loved ones. The manic energy feels great but is just not lasting as one does often experience some depression.

Another inspirational reading is by an unknown author:

The Power of Words

A careless word may kindle strife,
A cruel word may wreck a life,
A bitter word may hate instill;
A brutal word may smite and kill,
A gracious word may smooth the way:
A joyous word may light the day,
A timely word may lessen stress;
A loving word may heal and bless.

And, my favorites include a prayer by Sandra Pearse: Dear God, please give us the courage to let go of the thoughts and actions that would destroy us. Take control of our lives, for we will fall without you Amen.

And Psalm 37:5 Give yourself to the Lord: Trust in him and he will help you.

SUICIDE AND HELPING THE DEPRESSED PERSON

Often feelings of worthlessness, guilt and shame arise and the individual feels unfit to live. There is much pain and frustration during this process. Often, thoughts of suicide lead to actual suicides by someone who could have been saved by a caring loved one or friend. Suicide attempts will increase with advancing age.

However, suicide has increased in recent years among young adults as well as teenagers. Keeping this individual active and to feel useful is a first step. This individual should never be blamed for feelings of guilt or the depression itself. Depression should not be seen as a sign of weakness nor should one be told to snap out of it. Family or friends often compound the problem by blaming this often helpless depressed individual for his or her symptoms.

This depressed person is in serious pain and needs understanding and help. If the situation is prolonged, professional help should be sought. One thing to remember is that someone with only slight depression can attempt suicide.

Suicide is definitely not the answer. With the helpful understanding of family and loved ones, a good therapist and medication, all situations can improve. Sure, you are in pain, but consider the pain and suffering and often guilt you will put your loved ones, friends and family through if you follow through with suicide.

The following is one of the most inspiring poems I've ever read. I strongly urge you to type on an 8 X 10 paper and frame it by your front door, or by your dresser, and read it when you need such inspiration.

Don't Quit
by Edgar A. Guest

When things go wrong as they sometimes will,
When the road you are trudging seems all uphill,
When the funds are low and the debts are high,
And you want to smile but have to sigh,
When care is pressing you down a bit,
Rest if you must ... but don't you quit,
Life is queer with its twist and turns,
As everyone of us sometimes learns.
And many a failure turns about
When he might have won had he stuck it out.
 Don't give up though the pace seems slow —
You might succeed with another blow ...
Success is failure turned inside out —
The silver tint of the clouds of doubt —
and you can never tell how close you are,
It may be near when it seems afar.
So stick to the fight when you are hardest hit ...
It's when things get worse that you mustn't quit!

Remember, living on a roller coaster can be very exciting (highs) or very terrifying (depression), or you can even fall off. We build and plan our own lives and don't plan for the highs and certainly not the lows. With proper medical help, you can rebuild your roller coaster so as to enjoy the entire ride.

I have lived life on F A I T H (For After Intense Truth (is) Heaven.)

I have also survived on Hebrews 11 (1-16), Living Bible:

Another positive and strong message of revelation to me has been Matthew 10 (34-39). The Lord has been there my entire life, but obstacles of people have temporarily blocked our wave lengths. At these times, I have had to fight the good fight with all thy might. "In him I live and have my being." With God's help one can draw to himself the creative powers of the universe. We may stumble and we may fall, but we don't have to accept defeat. You must, however, be self-reliant and positive about God's power.

Manics are the most productive, creative, and successful work force in America. Manics control politics, Wall Street and the largest of all corporations. We are very gifted individuals, but we must avoid and also deal with depression. God put us on this earth lacking a body salt for a reason, so we could be great achievers and leaders. However, it takes strong, warm and understanding loved ones to understand us. My next wife will be an angel that the Lord, himself, has sent for me. I have, in fact, met six God-sent angels whose love and friendship and understanding I will always cherish. To Lucinda, Sandra, Susan, Marty, Sherry, and Donna, I have written this poem:

For some ... Life is full of hurt and pain

But with God's help and angels like you, we bounce back once again

I've had my failures but never defeat Because with hearts like yours, I feel, Keep me in the passenger's seat....

And, God at the wheel.

There may have been a lot of hate and anger released in this book.... But, that's just it.... I have released and dealt with it, and have no further resentment.

Poems of

James O. Wessinger III

To My Loving Children, Stacy and Jason
Written While Hospitalized and Afraid of Losing His Children's
Love

To Love is To Care
To Love is To Share
To Love is To Call
But by no means All
To Love me is to understand
And not to label me a certain brand
The only thing medically wrong with my brain
Is that it is faster than a speeding train
If you don't understand me then let me know
But don't as you have, let your love cease to show
I miss the good times we once had :
For I only want to be your loving Dad
The two of you could give me some love and support
For lately it falls much to short
This poem is not to make you feel bad
But only to stress the needs of your loving Dad
I really don't mean to make a fuss
For all I want is a genuine love between us
If it doesn't happen, then I'll disappear
For to be without love is worse than fear
If the two of you decide to let me go
Then these are two things I want you to know
For my love for you will never cease to grow
But it will be a love I hope I'll never know
I apologize for any stress and strain
All I want is your love and support once again
Since I was sixteen I have not lied
However, from the lack of your love, I have often cried
To continue without it, a part of me will surely have died.
Please call and write,
Your Loving Dad,

Roses are red and roses are yellow
Don't give up on me,
I'm a damn good fellow.

For some... Life is full of hurt and pain,
But with God's help and angels like you,
We bounce back once again.
For I had my failures, but never defeat,
Because with heart's like yours, I feel,
The Lord in the passengers seat....
And, God at the wheel.

I am so glad we are reunited.
I offer my love to bring,
You happiness and keep you excited.
Our love will be fresh as spring.
I no longer sit alone,
For I have so much planned,
And reservations to make a stand.
I love you so much today,
And I'm sure I'll love you more tomorrow.
I love you more than words can say,
And my strength is yours to borrow.
I offer you no pain,
Or a life full of booze.
For the world is yours to gain,
With nothing to lose

I can look you in the eye,
And my head begins to feel lighter.
I often wonder why,
But my whole life is just brighter.
I'm glad there is no other guy,
To compete with, because
I'm a fighter,
For your love I will not stand by.
For my life has been edited,
But please don't fret.
It's love from you for which I am credited,
And you will have nothing to regret.
For I offer you my love,
Because you are the nicest woman I've met.
And for you I offer the stars above..

Right now all I feel is emptiness,
For without you I am blue.
When I think of the things I miss,
It's not only you,
For it's your soft kiss.
Our love was beginning to be strengthen,
And from you I would take a life time sentence.
Now it only needs to be lengthen,
And for you III offer my repentance.
I'll sing for you at the top of my voice.
With me you can not lose,
Just make me your first choice.
You have just got to choose.

I only wonder what went wrong,
I just miss you so,
And I think of you almost every song,
For I hate to see you go.
When I first met you, you were a blast,
It felt so good to hold you tight.
If only our love could last.
I still think of you day and night

Please let me give my heart a try,
For I promise I will never deceive you or lie.
For in my love you will find,
A happy heart and a healthy state of mind.
I offer you love times seven,
And life as if it were heaven.
My love is only to satisfy,
And our love will surely multiply.
With these words, I do express,
And only hope your answer to them is yes

My love for you has already been told,
For it's a love that's twenty-fold.
Now I've got a lot of pride,
That's why I want you by my side.
I need you to keep my life on track,
For without you, my life is gloomy and black.
I set you on a pedestal above,
Just hoping to be worthy of your love.
Please don't let my heart be killed,
For all my love for you will not be revealed.

What in the world can I say,
to bring your love my way.
I'll love you in sunshine and rain,
for you I'll have fortune and gain.
I will love your heart and soul,
to get your love is-my #1 goal.
My love for you is lasting and long,
my love for you could never be wrong.

To gain your love would be a love story,
it would be one of riches, love, and glory.
Without you its hard to go to sleep,
I lay there trying not to weep.
As I sleep you're in my dreams,
filled with lakes, rivers, and streams.
For me you are the one,
Without you there is no fun.
I'm not ready to forget you yet,
for my heart just won't forget.

Take my heart and let it ease,
send your love if you will please.
Without you, I'll be low and down,
without your love, I'm a lonely clown.
The day you left me, my heart was shaken,
don't leave me this way, heartbroken and forsaken.
With these words my down payment is paid,
so please don't let your love be delayed.

I'd offer you the stars above,
but all I can offer you is my love.
I'm warm and caring, loving and sharing.
You can send me to the moon,
if you would just say" I love you " soon.
I want to satisfy,
for then our love can only multiply.

I can offer you the skies,
for your beautiful blue eyes.
I promise you well stay on top,
and our love will never stop.
To my love if you would just say yes,
then our love would never cease to express.
I'll love you more,
than there are sea shells ashore.
when you talk I'm all ears,
Let's let it last for the rest of our years.

"Let It Be Me"

To help you along the way,
for your love to stay.
Give me a chance to try,
for I'll promise III never lie.
We'll spend time together,
for there is nothing we can't weather.
Let me know if I go to fast,
because I want our love to last.
There's not much you don't know,
in time our love will show.
There isn't much I haven't told,
but I assure you my love is strong and bold.
I don't want my words to have too much power,
for I don't want this relationship to sour.
Don't muddle your thoughts with your mind,
let's see what our minds find.
I'll give you your space,
for this certainly isn't a rat race.
I'll take it day by day,
and hope your love will find its way,
for I want a love that is here to stay,
so dish it out if you may.
I hope your love for me hasn't got the slows,
because I want to make love to you before it snows.
Now my love for you has been revealed,
so the ball is in your field.

Roses are red and roses are white,
believe me darling I don't bite.
Roses are red and roses are yellow,
well my dear you have made me one happy fellow,
roses are red and violets are blue,
my dearest, I couldn't do without you.
I think of you first morning light,
I think of you noon and night.

Oh how I love you,
let me count the ways,
I love you more than there are docks in the bays.
I wish we just had time together to say,
words of how we feel and care.
For me your life is an open book to share.
To be away from you and your life,
would just bring about a lot of strife,
because one day I'm going to want you to be my wife.
My love for you is so strong,
therefore I can't be wrong.

We may have some failures,
But never defeat.
Because with hearts like ours,
I feel, will keep us in the passenger seat,
and God at the wheel.
Darling you are the sunshine of my days,
in fact I couldn't begin to count the ways.
I love you more than the sky is blue
I love you because of the lady in you!

When I woke up this morning I was feeling down and bad,
because I wasn't thankful to God for what I had
so when you need an uplift,
just remember, your gears may need shifting,
for the Bible reads "A man's mind leads the way.
But the Lord directs you" through your day,
S0, if you are down and troubled about a thing,
I suggest you go to the woods and sit by a river or spring,
ask yourself lately if you thanked God for his wonderful things.

I hope you brought your Bible,
cause you will be the one held liable,
God doesn't like one's Bibles to lay around with dust on it.
So each day read it if only a little bit.
Read it when you are up, read when down,
and read it when you're nothing but a silly clown.
When someone to you is mean and curt,
don't turn around and treat them like dirt.
Give a quote from the Bible and hope that's enough,
and maybe the rest won't be so rough.
The Bible teaches that one must have soul,
and a living and sensible goal.

Don't let your life be of anger and steam,
but one of a life long and a many of short dream,
At times you may feel your hands are tied,
but God is everywhere- We just need the patience of job.
Because God has never lied.
As he has given over 7,000 promises he'll keep.
For all his lost sheep.
You ask the reason I know,
I just have to open my Bible to show.

F For
A After
I   Intense
T Truth
H Heaven

"My Treasure Chest"

There are many truths that have been told,
there are many truths printed in bold.
Some things just grow still,
as they always will.
For we can have fun together,
in most any weather.
You see we are a chosen few,
for we are God's people nothing new.
For you see it's all told in your treasure chest,
which is your Bible and I call it your best.

When you read your Bible you start your shimmer,
but when you set it down you start to glimmer.
You realize that you saw the light,
and oh how simple and bright.
To me my bible is so dear,
because with it I have no fear
the Lord offers us his hand,
for which we all can stand.
I may have a lot of pride
but after all God is on my side.

It may take a while 'till I am a prisoner no longer
but God, Christ and me will hold out and just be stronger.
To come in here I didn't make a scene
for on the outside the pasture is more green,
and yet there are many things I haven't seen.
There are many things I have to do yet,
and God is my memory bank and won't let me forget.
The time to plant is NOW!
so get your plow!
I have been dealt some pretty ugly cards the last ten years
but with my faith in Got I have no fears.

They say it's all in my head,
but it's a pain in my heart instead.
They won't let me be me,
or consider setting me free.
For they are holding the card,
that I don't regard.
They say they just want more
I think more than there is sand on the shore.
However III last longer,
and come out stronger.
All this suffering from family and doctors was wrong,
for ten years is just entirely too long.
They don't have to be so curt,
and treat me like a piece of dirt.
Lately I've had tears like rain,
but once again I want some fortune and gain.
Until that comes,
I'll carry the load, up and down any road.
My enemies think they are so bright,
but they are far from right.
For my life I want again a natural feeling,
that will go straight through the ceiling.
Well God is number one in my life,
that will leave me from this strife.

Today I sit in sorrow,
awaiting a new and better tomorrow.
God, Christ, and me, we understand,
that some people aren't honest in this land.
Into her eyes I did stare,
Knowing she didn't have a care.
I rather be where the green grass grows,
for I'm no harm to anyone,
and everybody knows.
I get in trouble because I love my kids so much,
and this quack doctor makes it a six month crime for such.

Lonely

What do you do when you're sad and lonely,
first off don't think you are the one and only.
At first you may not have a human to care,
so first go to the lord and give him your prayer,
and you will find all of them he will bear.
Praise him in all spirits, tell him how you feel,
if you're depressed or happy you want to do his will.
The Lord is the king and no beginner,
He handles everyone in him and you can become a winner,
in the cold or in the hot of the sun,
your master should always be friend number one.
So praise him in all spirits and tell him how you feel,
if your depressed or happy you want to do his will.

Dreams

Dreams can be great,
they give us something to cling to,
but the bible says don't tary or be late.
And to begin from your dream is all up to you.
They often have talents of creativity,
but some people want face reality,
Dreams can cause a change in your life,
and even make a man take on a lovely wife.
Some dreams maybe scary and wrong,
while others bring about a song.
Some dreams make us cry,
while some make our thoughts fly.
Sometimes your dream may trouble your mind,
 but with a little change can make a mark on time.
The Bible says one should never stop dreaming,
or your life will just stop beaming.

I sit looking across this lonely field,
once again, my life to rebuild.
To rebuild from all the hurt and pain,
and to get on the top once again.
I just can't understand why,
some people want to see me cry.
For I'm not worried about a tear,
much less am I concerned about the fear.
For it says " Fear Not " 365 times in the Bible,
and after all God is holding them liable.

For My Daughter

Oh how I love you
Let me count the ways
I love you more
than there are docks on the bays.
I love you more,
I wish we just had time together to say,
words of how we feel and care.
For you my life is an open book to share.
I offer you only the truth without a lie
but to be away from you and your brother's life
often makes me cry
And without you two it just brings about more strife,
I am so proud of your achievements,
and ahead are only more accomplishments,
The price to pay is hard and some mistakes,
but I hope you learn from your heartaches.
You may have some failures
but never defeat,
I'll always feel,
if you keep the lord in your passengers seat
and God at the wheel.
And darling you are the sunshine of my days
in fact I couldn't begin to count the ways.
Remember, to love is to care
and to love is to share,
to love is to call,
but by no means all.
I love you more than the sky is blue,
I love you more because of the lady in you
Happy birthday and I love you more
than words can say.

Your loving dad who needs you.

With a lot of work and inspiration,
You have reached your day of gratification.
For it is your day of graduation.
Your work took you thousands of hours,
As does the beauty of growing flowers.
I've tried to show you love and affection,
But most of all a sense of direction.
Your education is something you planned,
Now you have something on which to stand.
Your work has been edited,
And now your life will be credited.
I offer you support and care,
And a true love to share.

I offer you a lifetime to share,
And it makes a lot of sense.
I offer you warmth, love and care,
So let me be your prince.
To show my love I sent you flowers,
With them I sent my affection.
But what I want is a love that's ours,
And a sense of direction.

I want a love that is caring and strong,
And for you I will be there.
I want a love that will last longer than long.
For III think of you when I say a prayer.
My love for you could never be wrong.
I offer you love and affection,
And I have a plan for us I'll explain,
Along with a sense of direction,
For we will work things out in times of sunshine and rain.

For you I would send a rose or daisy,
And they will need water and air.
And for your love, I am head over heels crazy.
I asked that your love be sent to me in a prayer.
My love, warmth and caring I send,
Knowing we are a perfect pair.
There is not a problem we can't mend

You are the sweetest lady I have ever met,
And on my list, you are on the top.
And my love for you,
I will never regret,
Nor will my love for you ever stop.
I love you so much baby,
If you'll just be my wife
Or at least say maybe.

If I'm coming on too strong,
I can come on a little lighter.
Because I want our love to be bold and long,
For I will make your life a lot brighter.
I'd rather have you near,
Than be out with a guy,
Drowning myself with beer,
Only to ask why.

At other women,
I will not stare,
For I want your heart,
And love to share.
Along with a commitment not to part,
With you I don't want to take a chance,
And with my love III never be late.
For I want our life to be one long dance,
And a love to share that will always be great

Darling

I love you from the first morning air.
I enjoy looking in your pretty eyes,
Knowing we are a perfect pair.
I know in choosing you, I was very wise.
And I love you noon and night,
For I know our love is right.
I'll make you like one of roses and daisies,
Because for you, I'm down right crazy.

To whom am I fooling,
I can't live without you baby.
I didn't know what I was doing.
I just lost my head maybe.
I want you to guide me in the right direction.
I know anger and love don't mix.
And I'll offer you love, warmth and affection.
There is no problem - we can't fix.

Darling you are so charming.
I think of you at my time prayer.
My love for to is bold and alarming,
I feel you will always be honest and fair.
I offer you the stars above,
But I don't want to move to fast.
Because I want your love,
And a relationship that will last.

I am sitting here with a broken heart,
Ever since you decided to part.
I can't believe we are through,
Because I still love you.
Why did our love have to ravel,
I was looking forward to romance and travel.
Our love could have reached the top,
And there was no reason to just stop.
Each night I say in a prayer,
That someday you will care.

I would walk many a mile,
Just to see your smile.
When you left, you didn't explain,
Why you left me in the rain.
Into your eyes I could stare,
And offer you love, warmth and care.
I long to hear your voice,
For I wish you would make me your choice.

My phone sits on the wall,
Waiting for you to call.
At night I sit looking in the sky,
Wishing I had you eye to eye.
As I stare and look above,
I wonder what happened to our love.
Without you my world is black,
I need you back to get on track.

God is my strength.
God is my guide.
He stays with me at any length,
And is always by my side.
I continue to read my bible.
And with God I feel on top.
The commandments for which I'm liable.
For I know my life will never stop.

I love you more than the sky is blue.
I love you morning, noon and night.
I love you so becasue of the Lady in you.
I love you first morning light.
To be without you—Juat wouldn't be right.
You remind me of a beautiful flower.
I just want o be with you everyhour.

I'll made my love for you very clear.
Yo lose you will be no duty.
My love and my heart will always be near,
For you are a thing of beauty.
You are the cream of the crop.
I love you so — this I know,
With you, I'm alays on top.
I love you more than I can show.

Happy Anniversery

With a lof of work and inspriration,
The tow of you have reached a day of gratification,
Your devoiton took thousands of hours,
As does the beauty of growing flowers.
The tow of you have showed love and affection,
But most of all a sense od direction.
We are so glad you are united,
Your love and happiness keep us exicted.
You will love each other more tomorrow.
Your sterngth is ours to borrow.
You love each other in good times and pain,
For the world is yours to gain.
You have offered each other all your love,
And the Lord offers you the stars above.
Your love is something you planned,
For now you have something on which to stand.
The Bible says your life has been edited,
And for sure you lives ill be credited,
We offer you support and care,
And a true love to share.
Happy Anniversery!

My Wonderful Son

I am so happy to now have custody of you,
You find it hard to chose between work and play,
You made my sun shine bright and my skies blue.
But just watching you makes my day.
Now that you have cleared up your foul mouth,
You are one of the biggest loverboys in the sough.
I have almost always taken your side,
With a Dady's joy and pride.
If you ut it to your mind,
The knowledge you need is in school to find.
With you I will always be fair,
I only ask from your time to share.
You have learned better to watch your temper,
And ?? to express.
And thus my answer will probably be yes.
With you here our love will only strenghten,
Like a lightning rod reaching to the ground to lengthen.
When you fell you need air,
Don't dispair.
Just remember I care.
You are not a boy any more, but a man,
So just remember to ask God fro help when you can.

Your Loving Dad.

My love for you is alarming,
I just hope I can stay as charming.
With the Lord and you I never feel alone,
I can always talk with you if only on the phone.
I look you in the eye,
And I wonder why,
You made me your choice.
I beleave our love is on the right course.

When we look together in a mirror,
Things seem so much clearer.
because our love is a beautiful sight,
Morning, noon and night.
I will love you through thick and thin,
And surely our relationship will win.
One day I may ask you to wear a wedding ring,
With all the lasting love that it will bring.

With you my heart begins to thunder,
I don't doubt your love for me or ever wonder.
With not harsh words to be spoken,
I don't think our love could ever be broken.
Of your love I have had a taste,
And I don't want it to go to waste.
With you I feel like I am on a mountain top,
Praying to God that our live will never stop.

My love for you flies high like an eagal,
And Ill'd do most anything for you that's legal.
Your love takes me of the ground,
And sometimes sends me heaven bound.
With you I know I can open any door,
Or walk along any shore.
In time our love will show the way,
And I am sure we will have happy days.

Lord, on this special day,
Let me take time to pray.
We thank you for the sky of blue,
We thank you for what you have us do.
We're so thankful for the sunshine, too,
And we ofer all our love to you.
For today is a special day to care,
As well as a special time to share.
Your love is worth more than gold,
Fore it cannot be bought or sold.
Now your love for us has been revealed,
And the ball is till in our field. Amen!

Dear Friend,

How are you? I just had to send a note to tell you how much I care about you.

I saw you yesterday as you were talking with your friends. I waited all day, hoping you would want to talk with me, too. I gave you a sunset to close your day and a cool breeze to rest you and I waited. You never came. It hurt me, but I still love you because I am your friend.

I saw you sleeping last night and longed to touch your brow so I spilled moonlight upon your face. Again, I waited, wanting to rush down so we could talk. I have so many gifts for you! You awoke and rushed off to work. My tears were in the rain.

If you would only listen to me! I love you! I try to tell you in blue skies and in the quiet green grass. I whisper it in the trees and breathe it in colors of flowers, shout it to you in mountain streams, give the birds love songs to sing. I clothe you with warm sunshine and perfume the air with nature scents. My love for you is deeper than the ocean, and bigger than the bibbest need in your heart!

Ask me? Talk with me! Please don't forget me. I have so much to share with you!

I won't hassle you any further. It is YOUR decision. I have chosen you and I will wait.

I love you!
Your friend,
Jesus.

                                                    Author unknown

To: My darling Stacy
  For today is your special day.
For it's your 21st Birthday.
And our recent past or land of doesn't matter such,
Fore I have so much to say.
But it all boils down to is that I Love You so much!
Please don't ever say good-bye to me again.
For it's only your love and support that I want to win.
To just drop me a little line or an inexpensive call would once
again me my feelings stand tall.
  That's not asking to much at all.
What I want is your unconditional Love,
It would mean to me, as much as the stars above.
To you I would never lie.
But, without your unconditional Love, it has often make me cry.
For I want to cry happy tears,
For my remaining years!

I Love You so much,

Your Dad.

REFERENCE NOTES

(1) *Mood Swings* - by Dr. Ronald R. Fieve, M.D.
(2) *Depression* - What We Know - National Lnstitute of Mental
    Health - Brana Lobel and Rober M. A. Hirschfeld, M. D.
(3) *Current Biographies* - 1979
(4) *Encyelopedia of Americana* - 1987, by Grolier Inc.

To order additional copies of this book, please send $19.95, includes tax, shipping and handling. For orders of three copies or more-$17.95 each. Rush delivery with money orders.
Please send your check or money order to:

Wessinger Foundation
P.O. Box 94
Thomasville, GA   31799

•••NOTES•••

•••NOTES•••

•••NOTES•••

190

•••NOTES•••

•••NOTES•••

•••NOTES•••